Facelift
Without
Surgery

J. B. Lippincott Company / Philadelphia and New York

Facelift Without Surgery

A 4-POINT PROGRAM TO MAINTAIN A YOUTHFUL FACE

by Ruth Jody

with Vicki Lindner

●

Copyright © 1979 by Ruth Jody and Vicki Lindner
All rights reserved
First edition
9 8 7 6 5 4 3 2 1
Printed in the United States of America
Published in association with Diane Harris

Photography: J. S. Zand
Drawings: Robert Handville

U.S. Library of Congress Cataloging in Publication Data

Jody, Ruth.
    Facelift without surgery.

    Includes index.
        1. Middle-aged women—Health and hygiene.
2. Face—Care and hygiene.   3. Beauty, Personal.
I. Lindner, Vicki, birth date, joint author.
II. Title.
RA778.J59   613'.04'244   78-21474
ISBN-0-397-01313-2

To my mother,
Rose Kolberg—
the prime mover

Contents

I would like to thank Professor William Linn for his constant encouragement and advice.

Vicki Lindner and I would like also to thank Berenice Hoffmann for her generous help with this project.

—RUTH JODY

Facelift Without Surgery

1 *Introduction*

When you're born your face is unformed; it is almost impossible to detect the features and expressions that will one day distinguish you as a unique individual. Babies and children are beautiful primarily because they're babies and children. At twenty you are dependent on youth and a fortunate genetic inheritance for your looks. As you grow older, however, your face becomes a mirror of what you have done, seen, felt, and thought, your habits and your state of health. Your passions, interests, and moral character register in the planes of your face; the expressions of your eyes and mouth are permanently etched in the skin around them. Triumphs, disappointments, frustrations, and delights settle in grooves we call "smile lines" and "frown lines." Your habitual moods communicate themselves without a word. You have created your own face.

Unfortunately, many of us dislike the face we have created, and we lump the markings of a rich and full life under the pejorative term "aging." The first wrinkle is for most of us a cause for panic, and we pray it is a temporary illusion some magical formula will be able to spirit away. When these lines become deeper and our skin begins to sag, we feel that youth and, with it, beauty have passed. We are soon to be old, we fear, and in the back of our minds *old* is synonymous with *ugly*. Anyone who is not young and smooth-skinned, we assume, is judged by our society as much less attractive than those who are.

Most of us accept this unfair cultural verdict. As we approach and pass forty, we feel we have reached the pinnacle of our lives. We may enjoy prestige, perspective, and great personal happiness, yet at exactly the point when we should rejoice that our faces reflect the full measure of our complex lives, we secretly regard ourselves as unattractive creatures. Some of us struggle to conceal the signs of advancing years and consider the words "You don't look your age" the supreme compliment. Others feel defeated by the symptoms of age and, after a certain point, do little to improve their physical selves. Who's going to look at, me? they think. But whether we greet the second half of our lives with equanimity or despair, none of us really believes it is possible to age beautifully.

AGING BEAUTIFULLY

I am convinced it is possible to be beautiful long past the age of forty—not just "presentable" or "acceptable" but truly attractive, elegant, and radiant with a sophisticated vitality. In Europe, where I was born, a chic older woman has always been the epitome of allure. Europeans recognize the fact that beauty is present not only in a smooth, unlined face but in a face that expresses a range of experience as well. A beautiful woman's face, they know, reflects her vital, interesting life, her enthusiasm for the activities she enjoys, and the subtle emotions she has felt.

If Europeans have a more positive cultural attitude toward the older woman, it is probably because she has a more positive attitude toward herself. Although the European woman, like her American counterpart, scarcely relishes the arrival of wrinkles, she knows they do not signify the decline of her sex appeal. She knows how to accept her age and make it work *for* her instead of against her. She is not considered chic simply because she is older, but because she grooms herself impeccably, using makeup, elegant clothing, and jewelry to express her unique qualities. She never gives up, when she reaches the middle of her life, or views her efforts to improve her appearance as a losing battle. She works hard to maintain a lithe silhouette, excellent skin, and vibrant good health. She is well aware that beauty after forty is not an accident but a job, requiring exercise, diet, skin care, and personal grooming.

WHAT IS A BEAUTIFUL OLDER FACE?

If aging were only a spiritual task, all of us who have lived vital, interesting lives would age beautifully. Our faces would mirror a fascinating life history, still in the making, and would be attractive to everyone. An older face, however, expresses the sum and substance not only of our psychic lives but of our physical lives as well. A beautiful older face is, by all cultural standards, a face which reflects good physical health. The lines and wrinkles exist, but the skin itself is still smooth, taut, and elastic. A beautiful older face is a slender face, with healthy skin and bright, lively eyes. In fact, a beautiful older face is only a more expressive version of a beautiful young face—robust and glowing with health and vitality. Health and vitality, however, come easily only to the young. As you get older, nature makes you work hard for them.

WHY WE AGE

Though age provides us with the positive benefits of wisdom and experience, it indubitably creates negative conditions in our bodies. These conditions begin long before we actually experience their results—soon after we've grown to our full physical size.

Briefly, the aging of the body is caused by the death of some cells in body tissue and the reduced functioning of the remaining cells. Cells shrink and atrophy as the body tissue they create functions less. Because we function less as we age, the cells atrophy, and because they atrophy we function less—a vicious circle. Brain and heart cells deteriorate, and hormones, which keep our skin soft and supple, slowly cease to be produced.

Another destructive process known as "cross-linking" is also responsible for aging. Cross-linking is the coupling of any two large molecules within or without the human cell; these molecules clog body tissue, causing its proteins to lose elasticity. The cross-links prevent the cellular regenerative substance, DNA, from doing necessary repair work. Gravity, too, is an enemy of youth; it pulls the soft tissues of the body downward for an unlovely sag. Heredity also affects aging, as surely as it does the formation of our features. People with long-lived parents live longer; people with parents who remained younger longer may be blessed with the same fate. Sunlight, artificial heating, pollution, and stress all conspire to age you.

Paradoxically, however, there is no scientific way of determining chronological age. Some people age earlier than others; presented with any two individuals who exhibit equivalent evidence of aging, there is no test of any kind which allows the scientist to say who is younger. Thus we arrive at the scientific basis for the two most common clichés about aging: Aging, alas, is inevitable, and you are as young as you look and feel.

HOW TO AGE: YOU HAVE A CHOICE

Given these facts, there are two ways to approach the aging process. We can accept our culture's negative idea that any face minus the full bloom of youth is automatically unattractive and resign ourselves to this unhappy destiny, neglect our external selves, and let our depression about aging affect what we do and how we think. Or we can simply accept the fact that we are older, realistically appraise the problems (and advantages) involved, and do all we can to make the situation agreeable.

If we want to age beautifully we must continue to develop emotionally, spiritually, and intellectually. We must stay involved in the activities we have always enjoyed and plunge deeper into life than we did before. We must also realize that to be an attractive older person is a physical challenge as well, a challenge we can either accept or ignore.

In short, we can become old and miserable about it as rapidly as possible, or we can take up the gauntlet and slow down the physical aging process. We can make our age work *for* us or against us. We can allow our external presence to mirror advancing disintegration or a vigorous, active life-style. We must realize that to age beautifully is a choice we make, preferably sometime before we are actually old—a choice which demands the development of disciplines and health habits that will help our bodies and faces remain beautiful throughout our lives.

WHAT IS A "FACELIFT WITHOUT SURGERY"?

To age well you must recognize before you are forty that your body, at forty, will not be the same self-restoring, efficient machine it was at twenty. The aging body has different needs and rhythms from the younger body, and poor health habits etch themselves quickly and permanently on an aging face. To cope with your "new" older body you must prepare yourself for an uphill struggle and hard work.

A facelift without surgery, then, is a system of exercise, healthful eating habits, and skin care that ideally should become part of your daily routine long before you find your face in trouble—the sooner in life you begin work on your "lift," the longer it will last. Whatever your age and physical condition, however, I guarantee you will become more vital and attractive once you make the habits and exercises I recommend a permanent part of your life. The sooner the better.

Basically, a facelift without surgery involves four interrelated disciplines: (1) facial exercises, (2) regular physical exercise, (3) diet, and (4) skin care. Although the facial exercises deal most directly with the signs of physical aging, they will not suffice by themselves. As a practicing rehabilitation therapist, I firmly believe that beauty is the expression of a positive spiritual and psychic condition as well as a physical state. To me, a face torn by anxiety, hatred, and disappointment is never beautiful, no matter how fresh and unlined the skin. Remember, aging beautifully is a total project which involves both the body and the mind.

Facial exercises

The main focus of *Facelift Without Surgery* is a set of isometric exercises I developed to move, tone, and firm the muscles of the face. Often, what we consider to be an unattractive aspect of an aging face—loose, sagging skin—may be the result of muscles beneath the skin shrinking and atrophying from lack of movement. These shrinking muscles leave gaps between themselves and the skin; the skin, no longer supported by underlying muscle tissue, hangs. Because facial muscles are small and numerous, the gaps and sags they leave in the face as they atrophy are conspicuous. This condition is aggravated by the fact that skin tends to lose subcutaneous fat as it ages. When facial muscles are put into use, the cells within them swell, the muscles increase in size and buttress the skin above them, and the face becomes taut and elastic again.

My facial exercises will not instantly revitalize the muscles of your face. At least three months of regular practice is required before the exercises have the desired effect. Sweep out any secret thoughts that you can accomplish the goal in less time. You will, however, see encouraging results after the first three weeks.

To learn the exercises you will need several concentrated sessions of hard work in front of a mirror; once you master them, fifteen minutes of facial exercises a day is sufficient. You may do them, as I do, while waiting for elevators, taking a bath, or watching TV.

Regular physical exercise

Medical specialists in the field of aging tell us that regular exercise is essential for a long and healthy life. I have always believed there is a strong connection between physical and emotional senses of well-being. When people exercise they feel better, and when they feel better they look better. A vital, healthy glow comes to their complexions; their faces are relaxed, free of tension. There are various physiological reasons for this phenomenon. When you exercise, an increased supply of blood and oxygen is sent to the muscles and tissues of the entire body, including the brain. You feel more alive because physiologically you *are* more alive. Exercise can even lift you from the depressions that make your face stiff, wooden, and unattractive. The reason why is not easy to explain, but I believe that unused physical energies form "traffic jams" in our bodies which physical exercise gets moving again.

In *Facelift Without Surgery* I will suggest ways and reasons to incorporate physical exercise into your regular routine and give you several exercises that are especially useful for relaxing the face and neck.

Diet

As our bodies age they no longer require the same number of calories they did to keep growing. Once you stop growing, you need only the calories necessary to maintain bodily functions, and any extra intake is really a waste product, stored in the unattractive form of fat. Scientists say we should always weigh what we did at eighteen; if anything our weight should decrease slightly as we get older. A low-calorie diet, like exercise, is necessary for health and long life. Yet how many of us weigh the same at forty as we did twenty years ago? To maintain your weight as you get older, you must decrease your intake of food by as much as a third. Yet most of us eat more, rather than less, and then try to lose the extra pounds with crash diets that promise us slimmer figures—instantly! Crash diets leave wrinkles and sagging skin in their wake, and overeating creates a puffy, bloated look, a double chin, and a bone structure hidden by fat— none of which makes you look any younger.

We overeat for emotional reasons, not because we're hungry. Our minds and bodies fool us with false signs of hunger we must learn for the sake of our health and figures to ignore. In this book I will show that the emotional reasons which cause us to stuff ourselves can be counteracted if we submit them to the harsh light of logic. I hope to help you develop the attitude, as well as the eating habits, necessary to maintain a constant body weight—so important for a youthful face and figure. I will give you my special tricks for dieting and for fooling your body when it is fooling you. My system for losing weight is not easy, but it works.

Skin care

To a certain extent beauty *is* only skin deep, but the skin is deeper than many people think and must be cared for from within as well as from without. I will tell you how to nourish your skin from the inside and design an efficient system for keeping it clean and fresh. I will also give you my tips on how to prevent the skin from aging prematurely and my ideas on makeup for the mature face, plus a special Ruth Jody facial treatment.

All over the world people still hope that somewhere lies a mythical fountain of youth and that one teaspoonful in a glass of water will banish the signs of accumulated years. Countless dollars are spent on wrinkle-removing creams, injections of vitamins, gerovital and hormones, and other elixirs guaranteed to restore youth and potency. Americans, especially, are great believers in instant results. And now those who fear aging are offered another instantaneous cure—the surgical facelift.

The American Medical Association reports that in 1972 one million people in this country alone underwent cosmetic surgery, and that in a short time the number will reach one and a half million. Though many surgical procedures are available to alter the structure of the face and torso, the most popular is the complete facelift, which promises to restore a face to its youthful contours by smoothing away wrinkles and sagging skin. Why, you may ask, did I bother to develop a difficult and time-consuming system of facial exercises when I could have gone to a hospital and come out younger—instantly?

Though the medical profession assures us that a facelift is a relatively simple, effective, danger-free procedure, I am not totally convinced. Consider what actually happens:

The surgeon detaches the skin on the face and neck from the tissues beneath, stretches and contours the skin to fit them smoothly, excises the excess, and sews the face back together again, leaving small scars around the hairline and ears. Another operation, called a blepharoplasty, is done to remove creases and bags around the eyes. Although modern surgical expertise and antibiotics have much reduced the dangers of the facelift operation, allowing this procedure to vastly improve the self-images of many people, it is by no means an "instantaneous" transformation without pain or difficulties.

Complications are possible. If the surgeon nicks the tiny nerves beneath the skin, partial facial paralysis may result, lasting for weeks or months. Sometimes too much skin is excised, resulting in a face that feels too "tight." Other dangers are death of skin tissue, severe scarring, and infections. Although serious complications are rare, most people who have had facelifts complain of some pain or discomfort. Side effects of the blepharoplasty occur more often: they may include sagging eyelids, constant tearing, inability to close the eyes, and even temporary blindness.

The cost of a facelift is, for people of average means, another complication. The regular lift, plus a blepharoplasty, hospital and surgeon's fees inclusive, averages $5,000. This costly procedure doesn't last. Age returns to the face in five or ten years, sometimes almost immediately. The price of a facelift is then an extravagant $500 to $1,000 a year!

Finally, there's a limit to what this expensive procedure can do. Wrinkles are made smoother but not eliminated. The facelift has virtually no effect on frown lines, smile lines, or small wrinkles above the lip. There are other surgical and chemical means to deal with these lines, including the injection of small drops of silicone, but these methods often involve real discomfort or danger.

Doctors have told me that the most successful face-lifts are done on people whose faces are still relatively young. The "skinny" face, as opposed to the fat, old face, benefits most from cosmetic plastic surgery. People with high, well-defined cheekbones, few wrinkles, and elastic skin with little underlying fat are the best candidates for the lift. Those with heavily sagging, wrinkled, or leathery-textured skins can be improved, but not much. A facelift cannot be performed on anyone who is in poor health or much overweight, either. In short, you have to be in good shape for a surgical facelift to work for you—and getting in shape is not an instantaneous process.

I personally would never consider such a facelift. I am an absolute coward and simply cannot imagine checking into a hospital and exposing my body to a traumatic surgical process when I'm not ill. Since I'm a mover and a doer, I can't imagine refraining from my favorite exercises, even for a short time, or taking care not to move my face too much when I talk or laugh for fear of "stretching" my lift. But most of all, I wouldn't dream of removing the lines which my life has engraved in my face and replacing them with an empty ironed-out look. I prefer my own safe, free, nonsurgical method of retaining a vital, youthful, and fully expressive face.

HOW I DEVELOPED A "FACELIFT WITHOUT SURGERY"

In approximately the middle of my life I underwent a traumatic experience well known to one out of three married women—I was divorced. At the time of the separation I experienced what all women, whatever their age, must discover in that situation: I suddenly realized I was alone, the person I'd expected to be with for the rest of my life was gone, and I might never meet another man I could love. I felt depressed and unattractive. I cried through movies, both happy and sad. I talked to my friends—but how many times could I tell the same story?

In order to feel more attractive, I immediately began to diet. I lost weight and found that literally overnight my skin developed wrinkles and sags it had never had before. Apparently my "crash" diet had helped deplete the sub-cutaneous fat which was keeping my face firm and unlined. My expression, moreover, was wooden; my face looked bitter, angry, resentful. And then, of course, there were the new wrinkles and bags. I realized I had to do something about my appearance. I wasn't afraid of aging, but I wasn't about to sit back passively and watch my face become old in an ugly, unpleasant way. Fortunately, I was better equipped than most people to attack these undesirable signs. Exercise and gymnastics had always been an integral part of my life—thanks to my mother's influence.

At eighteen my mother shocked the Jewish community of Frankfurt by opening a gym studio. (This was almost sixty years ago, when in some people's eyes physical exercise for women was equal to prostitution.) At the same time she began to study with the great dancers of her time, Harold Kreutzberg, Rudolf von Laban, and Mary Wigman. Mother was convinced that sports, dance, and movement were as vital to life as oxygen. She had a talent for making people aware of how they moved their bodies; she helped her pupils become self-assured and graceful. As they studied with Mother they inevitably became beautiful—and *beautiful,* in Mother's terms, meant *skinny.* She zoomed in on her students' eating habits and screamed and scolded when they put on pounds. Even today, in her late seventies, she is notoriously tactless to overweight students in her gymnastics classes, which she still teaches with the same vigor. But her tactlessness reaps rewards; she drives people to get the figures they want by making them work hard.

I came to exercise as naturally as I came to speech. Mother began to exercise with me when I was only four months old. She held me by the legs and let me dangle. She let me walk on my hands. She put me in the water and floated me around, moving my arms and legs in all directions. I was no more than three when she had me stand at the back of her gymnastics class and hop along. At five I was enrolled in the Leslie and Kuhn School for Acrobatic Performers, where, as the youngest student, I learned tumbling, splits, flips, walkovers, and swinging from high bars.

She also forced me to accompany her on the Sunday *Spaziergang,* or walk, in the mountains, an activity I did not enjoy. I was usually cranky, hot, cold, hungry, or thirsty, but Mother insisted. As a kid I could run faster, jump higher, back bend farther, and do more somer- saults than anyone else. I had no fears. I instinctively knew that when I did a flip-flop, I would land on my feet. Those activities I learned as a child remained a vital part of my life; they taught me precision and control, pleasure in achievement, the will to work hard and get whatever I did right. Now, by the way, like most Europeans, I love to walk.

When we came to New York during the Hitler era, many of Mother's gymnastics clientele came too. She used our apartment as a studio, and my first memories of New York consisted of half-clad women jumping about and piles of clothes in all the rooms. Irate neighbors rang our doorbell and banged on the ceiling. Thus, gymnastics became an inescapable part of my life in America too. But it was soon apparent to me that, as much as I liked exercise, it could never become my whole life. I entered college and studied psychology.

Still, I never abandoned my devotion to my body or my delight in physical activity. I have studied ballet, modern dance, Tai Chi, Indian yoga, and the Russian dance, Kazatska. I swim, bicycle, play handball, jog, and jump rope. All movement—dance, sports, and mountain climbing—interests me. I've taught gymnastics and physical therapy in schools, hospitals, and camps my whole life. I often assist my mother in her gymnastics studio today.

Thus, when it came time to take drastic measures to restore my face, I immediately resorted to my gymnastics background and my deep sense of body. I felt that wrinkles and sags in the face were no different from those in other parts of the body; I was sure they were related largely to muscle inactivity. I read a book on facial exercises, but, my God, there were at least thirty-five of them with elaborate instructions. Busy people should not be expected to spend half the day exercising their faces, I thought. Moreover, there wasn't a word in this book about the effect on the appearance of diet, skin care, regular exercise, or psychic well-being.

I remembered the facial exercises I had seen during the summer of 1974 when my mother and I traveled to the Aslan Institute in Rumania to learn what the Eastern countries were doing about aging. They used only simple, traditional facial exercises, and it seemed that these were not enough. Then I examined a chart of facial muscles. I saw that many muscles in the face simply didn't do anything in the course of normal facial movements. Slowly, one eye on the muscle chart and the other on the mirror, I worked on my face. I found it challenging and interesting to discover ways to exercise muscles in my face that I'd never moved before.

Shortly, my face seemed less wooden and pasty looking. After three months there were visible results. When I touched it my skin was more resilient and elastic, less flabby, and it adhered more tightly to my bones. The wrinkles were smoother. In short, the exercises worked. My face looked and felt younger. I'd given myself a facelift, naturally, without the cost and medical trauma of surgery. I received innumerable compliments. "What did you do?" my friends asked. Some wanted easy answers, but others wanted to learn the exercises. I began to teach my facial exercises to these friends and to the men and women in my mother's gymastics studio. They worked, not only for me, but for others as well. A moderate diet, regular exercise, and periodic visits to a European cosmetologist were already part of my life routine. I wanted to encourage others to adopt my total system for health, vitality, and youth. The result is this book.

Your first question is predictable: "How old is Ruth Jody?" I leave my age to your imagination because, unlike so many people, I don't relish the compliment, "You don't look your age." I know that I look and feel terrific, and as they say in Europe, "What does age have to do with it?"

2 *Face It!*

Your face is the most visible part of your body, an open testimony to your emotions, moods, state of health, and, often, your age. Yet chances are you've never seen your own face. The face is the only part of our body we never see directly with our eyes. Although we can examine our hands, legs, bellies, and even, with a little neck craning, our backs, when someone says, "You have a smudge on your face," our fingers grope helplessly to find it. Thus, we must rely on mirrors for knowledge of our faces, but mirrors are deceptive reflecting pools. Why? First, mirrors cannot reveal us as we are because we unconsciously present a different face to the mirror than we do to the rest of the world; and second, most of us come to the mirror with an image of our face already fixed in our minds and never allow ourselves an honest, objective look in the glass.

The face we show to the mirror is generally designed to increase self-esteem. Most of us arrange a "special" face for the mirror. For the mirror we smile our most enchanting smiles, bask in the calm of the purest serenity. In times of trouble we compose our distraught features into an untroubled expression before exposing them to the looking glass. None of us, it seems, wants to see a face blasted by anxiety, sorrow, or anger. Think back to the last time you were upset. Before you went to the mirror, didn't you erase the unpleasant emotions from your face, smoothing it into a blank you found more acceptable? On less trying days we pose for the mirror much as we would pose for a camera. We set our features into what we consider their most attractive expression and look in the mirror as we wish to be seen.

Few of us, in any case, go to the mirror to see our faces as they are but only to beautify them—to shave, comb our hair, or apply makeup and creams. Our mirrors, too, are often illuminated by soft, flattering lights. We try to please ourselves by putting our best faces forward and providing an ideal reflection. As a result, few of us see the face that everyone else sees—fully animated, expressing the subtle range of emotions that passes through our minds in a variety of physical and psychic circumstances. For this reason we have all had the experience of surprising ourselves in a full-length display window or an unsuspected mirror lurking beneath fluorescent lights and exclaiming with horror, "My God, is that me?"

We react just as negatively to a photo we consider unflattering. When shown an unfamiliar, unpleasing portrait, most of us moan, "Is that the way I really look?"—

hoping for the reply, "Heavens, no, you're much better looking than *that*." We choose photographs for our scrapbooks that present a self-image we approve of—and the truth is, that image may bear little resemblance to our real selves. Although some photographs may indeed present a less ideal image than others, they may be more accurate than the ones we frame. I've often found my family and friends prefer photos of me which I hate; these pictures, they say, look more like me. In other words, the face they love is mine; the face I love exists mainly in flattering photographs and my imagination.

Actually, our image of how we look is formed before we confront ourselves in a mirror or photograph. The image we carry is an internalized one, buried deep inside ourselves. It has been formed by a vast number of judgmental messages we have received about our appearances since childhood from relatives and friends and has little or nothing to do with our real faces. These judgments arrived en masse in the form of critical appraisals, approving smiles, and flattery and their opposites— disapproval, childish insult, negative looks. Your mother's constant admonition, "You certainly go to school looking like a slob," your father's indication that to him you look like an older sister, only not quite as pretty, your brother's taunt, "Hey, beanpole!", your best friend's advice, "Why don't you straighten your hair?" and your grandmother's words, "You look like an angel, darling," all enter your psyche to form a confused picture of yourself—a skinny, slovenly, frizzy-haired angel.

Throughout our lives what people have said, forgotten to say, or silently implied about our external selves has been interpreted and stored, or misinterpreted and stored, as an internal photo of our faces and forms. As we grow older, this internal photo grows too—a muddy product of even more approving and disapproving reactions. The mirror, for most of us, only confirms the way we see ourselves in our mind's eye or creates additional confusion.

Take me, for example. When I was a child in Germany, I quickly learned that redheads with freckles were no one's idea of heavenly pulchritude. Freckles were nothing more than splotchy blemishes, and red hair was a blatant eyesore. Each night I spent hours carefully daubing each freckle with freckle cream, afraid to apply the cream to my whole face for fear of making the space between the freckles even paler. No one, but no one, ever said I was pretty. Later, I came to America and discovered that here redheads were sexy and exotic fare, but the damage had already been done. I hated my red hair and freckles with a passion that no new message of approval could entirely erase. When I looked in the mirror, part of me saw the glamorous redhead that was now "hot stuff" while another, deeper part saw the blemished, sharp-featured face of a homely schoolgirl.

Most of us maintain such confused images of ourselves. Our feelings about our faces change drastically with our moods. When we are rejected, bored, or angry, we feel ugly; when we are loved, admired, or praised, we feel beautiful, although our actual physical appearance has changed only minutely, if at all. If you were made to feel ugly when you were young, you will have to fight your whole life to feel beautiful, no matter how beautiful you become. Even Marilyn Monroe suffered this fate. And though most of us are not beautiful or ugly or extremely neurotic, few of us like our faces and most of us feel we are less attractive, in some way, than we are supposed to be.

The idea of how we are supposed to look is formed not only by what others say or do not say about our appearances, but by images of ideal beauty fed to us by the media throughout our lives. The ideal face, we are led to believe, is the one seen constantly in cosmetic ads, in fashion magazines, in movies, and on TV—a suntanned, flawless oval adorned with even, small, regular features. This ideal, often the product of makeup, flattering photography, or an airbrush, is always serene; it expresses no negative emotions. Few of us resemble it or know anyone who does.

We are surprised to recognize famous models or media stars in person and find that they are not especially beautiful at all; many of them look ordinary, uninteresting, or older and less vibrant than we expect. Still, our unconscious minds continue to uphold these faces as ideals. We compare our own, usually unfavorably, with them, even while our conscious minds reject them as "beautiful." Because while growing up we have been force-fed the idea that Rock Hudson, Shirley Temple, or Twiggy represents Beauty as it should be, we find these ideals permanently instilled in our unconscious. By the time we are old enough to form aesthetic opinions of our own, we are no longer capable of applying them to our own faces. We disown our faces and apply our real ideals of beauty to the people we know.

THE OLDER FACE

The ideal face we see in the media is, needless to say, always young. No beautiful faces past the age of forty are

Face It!
33

held up to inspire our sighs and swoons. How many of us actually believe there is such a thing as a *beautiful* old face? If an older face seems lovely, we are inclined to mutter the feeble compliment, "She must have been a great beauty in her day," or, worse, "She certainly is well-preserved." In other words, the wrinkles of "former" beauties are regarded as unnatural lines penciled in on a face that in all fairness should have remained eternally young, and we regard our own wrinkles the same way.

Our cultural standard of beauty throws no crumbs to the aging. When we are young we may feel unhappy that we will never look like Catherine Deneuve, but none of us is supposed to aspire to look like an aging Catherine Deneuve. When we are encouraged by the media to admire the appearance of an older person, it is usually someone extremely rich and soignée—Jacqueline Onassis, for example. Such people wear fabulously expensive clothes, are pampered constantly in high-priced salons, and, we assume, have well-done facelifts whenever necessary. Never, we feel, have they plunged their silken hands into dishwater or scrubbed a kitchen floor. Their money, in effect, is what keeps them well-preserved, and their images cause those anxious about aging even greater despair. Who can afford to look the way they do? In short, those of us who wish to maintain a positive image of the aging face are cultural pioneers.

DOUBLE STANDARDS

Although we may castigate ourselves because we don't have the right nose, the profile of a glamorous movie star, or the face of a twenty-year-old when we're forty, we would never dream of applying these same, admittedly ridiculous standards to the faces of our friends. None of us dwells on a slightly oversized nose, wrinkles, sags, or smile lines when they belong to the people we love. We would never dream of greeting an old acquaintance we met unexpectedly with, "My God, is that you?" When someone we care for starts looking "bad" to us, it's not because we have suddenly noticed less-than-perfect features or new wrinkles but because this person is in poor health, hung over, depressed, or angry.

Good looks and youth admittedly attract us to others, as do beautiful clothes and perfect grooming; but physical beauty creates only a temporary allure, and we have all had the experience of watching a beautiful or handsome face grow unpleasant when we discovered that person was stupid, dishonest, obnoxious, or cruel. Few people in the world are objectively truly ugly or beautiful. As we get to know others, their faces become attractive to the degree that we like or dislike their characters and personalities. Even if we find a certain pair of blue eyes enchanting, their charm will all but vanish if we cease to admire their owner.

We focus far more on our friends' expressions of emotion and thought than on the actual physical construction of their faces. We all know how much more beautiful a woman friend becomes when she's in love, although nothing has happened physically to change her. We see the glow of good health, peaceful relaxation, and sincere animation far more than a specific set of features. Nonetheless, when we look at ourselves we promptly fall victims to confused internal images and the artificial standards of beauty promoted by the media. The verdict ranges from self-love to self-hatred. We sigh and moan and wish for a different nose, a better head of hair, or a more youthful forehead. We wish the fictitious face we have in mind would materialize in the mirror, and this futile wish keeps us from ever seeing ourselves with the warmth, affection, and wholehearted approval that others do.

A facelift without surgery will improve your appearance in concrete, visible ways; facial exercises, if practiced regularly, will increase the elasticity and tone of your skin; regular physical exercise will bring you a vibrant color and a relaxed expression; diet will improve your health and facial contours; and proper skin care will also make a difference you can see. But my four-point system will be fruitless if, in the end, you are unable to look at yourself with a good measure of self-love. This self-love must not come from a vital change in your appearance, but from a more accepting attitude toward it. You must be willing to see yourself in a new way—as you are. Before you attempt my program, then, it is important to shed the distorting masks of negative value judgments which cause you to condemn yourself. How can you do this? By really looking at your own face.

I believe that when you take a long, objective look at your face, you will not, as you fear, see an uglier, more grotesque visage than you imagined, but a more acceptable version of yourself. As you rid yourself of double standards, false cultural images, and internalized visions of yourself, your real face will emerge before your eyes— older, yes, not beautiful but not ugly either, simply a face which belongs to you and no one else, the mirror of a unique history and a unique inner landscape. The longer and more realistically you look at yourself, the more you can identify with and appreciate what you see.

When you really look at yourself, you may find that obsessions with "bad" features have prevented you from seeing the better aspects of your face. For example, if you despise your wrinkles and see only the deep grooves etched from nose to mouth, you may be overlooking your beautiful eyes, determined chin, or sensual lips. On the other hand, an obsession with wrinkles may also prevent you from spotting flaws in your face that you might easily take steps to correct—a complexion pasty from lack of exercise or, one of the most common flaws, an unbecoming makeup job. Your unflinching focus on your wrinkles may prevent your eyes from traveling downward and noticing that you've gained five pounds.

When you view yourself objectively, you stop turning yourself off with unrealistic ideals. As you begin to accept, even admire, your own face, it becomes more possible for you to enjoy the efforts you make to beautify it, instead of regarding them as last-ditch rescue measures for a sinking ship. When I learned my divorce was final I decided to attack my doldrums with a stylish haircut. I liked myself better right away. I came home, took a pleased look in the mirror, then stifled my inclination to put on my prettiest dress and rush out to have lunch with a friend. "Wait a minute," I told myself, and took another look. I decided to go to Bergdorf's and have my eyebrows dyed.

Every time I looked, the more I liked myself, and the more I liked myself the more it became possible to pamper myself, to improve my face and take pleasure in doing so, instead of skimming over my reflection with a distasteful glance. The new haircut and eyebrow job

Face It!
37

probably scarcely changed my looks at all as far as my friends and children were concerned, but my image of myself improved, and I faced the world with a revitalized expression. Self-love, I discovered, can give you a bit of the glow another person's love gives you.

Even after you accept your own face, negative internalized images may return along with personal difficulties. As soon as you begin to feel unattractive, look at yourself again. When I'm burdened by heavy job pressures, I tend to envision my face as a heavy, dull mass, expressionless, like a robot's. Then I force myself to take a long, cool look in the mirror again. My first reaction is inevitably, "Hey, I still have red hair; I still have blue eyes. I look all right!"

Looking at yourself objectively and renouncing negative value judgments about your appearance will prevent you from indulging in the futile game of "I wish." The "I wish" game goes like this: You look in the mirror and see the horizontal wrinkles creasing your forehead. "If only I didn't have them; I wish I didn't have them; I shouldn't have them," you moan. You get stuck on those wrinkles— or your oversized nose or your hair or your freckles—and lose your ability to admire your face. The "I wishes" and "should and would haves" afflict you with anxieties that go nowhere. To say "I wish" is an admission that it's impossible to *do* anything, and the energy you spend saying "I wish" could be spent on productive activities. A facelift without surgery asks you to stop wasting good emotional energy on "I wish" and put that energy to work.

How, you may ask, can I look in the mirror and see a different face? At first, you may have to take radical steps to see yourself as you are. Here are some suggestions.

Discover your face

Before you look in the mirror, close your eyes and attempt to see your own face. You will probably find this more difficult than you suppose. You may, in fact, see a nearly blank oval, and the actual image of your features may elude you. Try to visualize the exact color of your eyes, the shape of your nose, lips, and chin, the position and shape of your eyebrows, the tone of your skin. Now, open your eyes and look in the mirror. With your eyes on your face, describe your features as you see them. Move from feature to feature and describe it as objectively as possible. Do not say, "I have a beautiful mouth" or "I have an aristocratic nose." *Beautiful* and *aristocratic* are value judgments—they do not tell you anything. Do not use metaphors (for example, "I have sea-green eyes"), or words which imply value judgments, such as "bent" nose or "sunken" cheeks. Do not approve, condemn, or romanticize; merely describe. Instead of "sea-green" or "beautiful" substitute "blue with yellow and brown flecks in the irises" for the color of your eyes. Instead of "big, crooked nose" say "a nose that widens at the tip and has a raised bone just below the bridge which curves slightly to the left."

Describe your bone structure, the color and texture of your skin, the shape and consistency of your eyebrows, even your wrinkles. If you can, describe the shape of your eyes and the fold of your eyelids. Use as many de-

Face It!
39

tails as possible. You will be astonished to discover how much you have to say about your face, how difficult it is to avoid value judgments, and how much more you are seeing than you usually do. Once you eliminate words like "beautiful, horrible, aristocratic" and other praise and condemnation from your description of yourself, you will be surprised to find how little these words actually mean and how much you have relied on them. When you've finished the mirror exercise, close your eyes and again try to visualize your face. You may find a much-improved image in your mind's eye.

Ask others to describe your face

This exercise takes more courage. Explain to your friends that the purpose of their description is not to flatter or reassure you, but to give you a better idea of how your face appears to those around you. Some people will decline, but those who accept may give you interesting clues about how others see you. You will certainly find that your friends don't dwell on your oversized nose, smile lines, or wrinkles. Instead they will reveal what makes you an attractive individual to them. You may find that your smile, the expression in your eyes, and other qualities you never considered at all enter their descriptions. It may be difficult for them to describe your face, not because they've never looked but because its essence is intangible to them.

If you think you can take it, ask your friends to describe what they find unattractive about your face. Again it may be an emotional expression, a "face" you make unconsciously, more often than a specific feature that makes a negative impression. It may even be your makeup job they dislike. You will discover from this exercise that your friends see different qualities in your face than you do.

Get rid of double standards

Before you disabuse yourself of double standards you must first become aware of what they are. Ask yourself which of your friends you find beautiful or attractive and why. What, exactly, do you consider attractive about them? Ask yourself the same question about famous people and about strangers you see on the street. Define what you consider interesting, dull, lovely, or repelling in a face. During theater intermissions examine the faces of women you find glamorous—do they have perfect oval-shaped faces, nary a wrinkle, or tiny, upturned noses? Find out exactly what it is about people's faces that you admire. What role do "intangible" qualities play in forming your opinion? What is it about a person's eyes or facial expressions that turns you on—or off? This exercise should make you aware that you apply different standards to yourself than to the people around you.

See your face in action

Darwin discovered that anger, grief, shame, and joy are expressed in the same way on people's faces in every culture. Your face is a remarkable reflector of your emotions; imagine how complex the nerves and muscles must be if they can so quickly portray what you feel. To learn how you really appear, then, you must see your face in action. Few of us laugh, cry, frown, think intensely, or look angry before a mirror, so we have little idea what we look like when we do. Unless we are masters of self-control, various indications of our moods and thoughts cross our features all the time, and it is these expressions that define our faces to others.

Try out your emotional muscles before the mirror: laugh, frown, smile, grimace. Think of recent situations in your life and try to reproduce your face as it was at those moments. If something made you angry recently, think about it and look angry. Think sad and happy thoughts, frustrated thoughts, and nostalgic thoughts, and notice how they change your face. Ask yourself which of these expressions appears most often on your face. Which of them strikes you as ugly or beautiful? Think furious thoughts, then deliberately compose your face. Do you find your expression natural or stiff and wooden? Next time you are really angry, look in the mirror. Let your anger show. You may be surprised to find you like an expression of real anger better than controlled anger. The next time you cry, do it in front of the mirror. You may feel silly at first, but you will find this exercise illuminating. You can practice it in public, too. Next time you're at a dinner party chatting with your friends, for example, sneak a look at yourself in the dining room mirror. Sneak looks at your face in action whenever you can.

3 *Facial Exercises*

We tend to think that wrinkles alone signify an aging face. The lines which furrow our cheeks and foreheads, however, are not the only reflections of advancing years. The most dramatic and conspicuous evidence of aging is, in my opinion, a loose and sagging face. The flabby skin beneath the jaw, a shrinking eye, slack cheeks, drooping corners of the mouth, a furrowed upper lip, and a "witch's" nose and chin with hanging tips are, to me, the least attractive hallmarks of age. These unpleasant specters are all results of atrophied muscle tone and simultaneous loss of underlying facial flesh.

As the body ages, the muscle structure beneath the face diminishes automatically; our faces lose the buttressing flesh that kept them taut and full, and gravity pulls the loosened skin downward. Although wrinkles are not necessarily unattractive, a sagging facial skin connotes inactivity and decrepitude. Both wrinkles and sagging skin are inevitable expressions of age and appear sooner or later, depending on skin type, hereditary tendencies, general state of health, exposure to the elements, and other factors largely beyond our control. Even though there's not much we can do to erase wrinkles, the slack muscle tone of the face can fortunately be tightened up again, like sagging muscles anywhere in the body, with exercise.

THE MUSCLES IN THE FACE

We imagine muscles as visibly bulging structures in the arms, legs, and back. Therefore, it is a surprise for many of us to learn that the face, too, is crisscrossed with muscles, although the facial flesh is smooth and soft. A glance at the facial atlas on page 56 proves beyond a doubt that there are as many muscles in the face as in any other part of the body—not tiny, insignificant muscles, but large and powerful ones. Only the temples, skull, and small spots on the chin and the center of the nose are totally without muscles. The facial muscles, moreover, are voluntary muscles, which means we can move them at will, unlike the involuntary muscles in our internal organs, over which we have no control.

That's not to say we *do* move our facial muscles. Some, like those we use to smile and chew, get a regular workout, but the majority of the muscles in the face never move of their own accord but are merely "pulled" along, like dead weights, when we make our habitual facial movements. Our eyes, for example, are ringed by powerful muscles, but when we open and close them, we use only the muscles in the upper lids; the muscles in the lower lids get pulled along. These inactive facial muscles

Facelift Without Surgery
44

can be compared to the muscles in our toes, which get a free ride from the muscles of our thighs and calves as we walk but never do any work of their own.

Some of the muscles in our faces have become so weakened by generations of nonuse that now it is almost impossible to move them at all—the auricular muscles, which can theoretically be used to wiggle the ears, for example. Sometimes we inadvertently put these lazy muscles into action, such as when we laugh so hard our faces actually hurt. That achy feeling is nothing more than our facial muscles reminding us that they exist. Whenever we put an inactive muscle to work any place in the body, it gets larger, fuller, stronger, and becomes more visible in the flesh.

Muscles are responsible for keeping the face smooth and soft. If we allow nature to take its course and atrophy the muscles as we age, the spaces between the muscle structure and the skin increase, creating loose skin and sags. On the other hand, if we learn to exercise the atrophying muscles of the face, they will increase in size and fill the gaps between the skin and the muscle itself. When the sagging skin is drawn taut again, wrinkles, too, are "ironed out" so that the face appears smoother.

A surgical facelift, as I have said, is done according to the same principle: The surgeon pulls the patient's sagging skin tightly across the face and excises the excess. However, this is only a temporary reprieve because the condition of the underlying muscles is not improved. As the muscles beneath the skin continue to shrink and cells of the buttressing flesh are lost, the skin stretches out again and the patient must return to the surgeon for another lift. Needless to say, any exaggerated movements made with the face—smiles, frowns, laughter—help to speed the skin-stretching process. If the surgical facelift were painless, cheap, and not traumatic, there would be no reason for those of us who dislike the effects of aging to bother with facial exercises. But for anyone who fears surgery and its difficult aftermath, or who cannot afford to spend $5,000 every time a surgical lift needs to be done, facial exercises are a viable and effective alternative.

MY SYSTEM OF FACIAL EXERCISES

Although exercising the face is a relatively new concept, it is certainly not unique. Exercise and gymnastics studios often teach facial exercises as part of a general body-toning routine, and there are several other books on the subject. Most existing facial exercise systems, however, are based on exaggerations of the expressions we usually make with our faces—grins, squints, and so on. These exercises are fairly easy to perform but accomplish little because they tend to exercise the muscles already in use.

My system teaches you to use different muscles to make familiar expressions and thus to exercise muscles in your face you've never used. Physical therapists teach stroke victims, whose muscle tissues have deteriorated, to perform their previous functions by allowing one muscle to take over the action of another. In the same way, you can learn to transfer energy from one muscle to another in your face, forcing the facial muscles that usually get dragged along to work and increase in size. For example, when you pout you usually use only the muscles of your lips, but if you relax your lips and make your cheek muscles do the work necessary to keep the lips in a pouting position, you have brought an entirely new set of muscles into play.

WHAT WILL FACIAL EXERCISES DO FOR YOU?

Shortly after you begin regular practice of my facial exercises, the muscle tone in your face will visibly improve. After three months of exercises, your skin will become more taut and your face will look smoother. These facial exercises will not only strengthen and fill out the muscles of your face but will also stimulate blood circulation, bringing new plasma into the small blood vessels there. As a result, your skin color and tone will improve, and your face will look and feel more animated, more alive. Compliments from friends are guaranteed. "How well you look!" is a refrain you can count on hearing over and again. You must not, however, expect the unlined, flawless face of your twenty-first year to magically reappear. You will look younger, but you will not look *young*. When you think about it, would you really want back again the bland face of early youth, minus the characteristics your individual life experience has put there? I know I wouldn't.

Once your face improves you will be inclined to relax and stop the exercises. *Don't!* Only regular and consistent practice of my facial exercises provides lasting improvement. Don't expect to do the exercises once or twice a week and see results or to stop doing them altogether and maintain their effects. You must practice facial exercises every day without fail if you want them to work. You may find, to your surprise, that you actually enjoy doing the exercises—especially when you begin to see their results.

Any accomplishment brought about by your own efforts is more gratifying than one that comes to you from the outside. Thus, you will find the effort you expend to create a firmer, younger-looking face benefits your psyche, too.

WILL EXERCISING THE FACE CAUSE WRINKLES?

As you do these exercises you will contort your face into positions which create temporary wrinkles. If I continue to do them, you may ask, will those wrinkles engrave themselves permanently in my face? The answer is no. The skin of the face is highly elastic, and it takes untold repetitions of a single expression to press a wrinkle into your skin.

Experts believe that the entire structure of the face is largely created by our emotions, which shape the muscles, planes, and features. Emotions affect blood circulation and even change the way our faces appear from day to day. I think that the wrinkles we find especially unpleasant are caused by negative inner thought patterns which habitually move the face into characteristic expressions. Disappointment, bitterness, tension, and anxiety result in the wrinkles we could all do without—deep frown lines between the brows and creases above the upper lip, for example. Smile lines on the sides of the mouth and crinkles at the corners of the eyes may betray your age, but they do not give out the unhappy vibrations that the lines caused by negative thought patterns do.

I've noticed that during difficult periods of my life, my wrinkles become deeper and more noticeable. My facial skin, too, feels flabby and looks sallow, as if tension were preventing the blood from reaching it. At times when I feel relaxed and content, my wrinkles by no means vanish, but they tend to fade. I've seen very young people with frown lines and very old people without any at all. Therefore, I've concluded that it is not age per se that produces those especially unwanted lines, but the years of disturbed psychic feelings that a face reflects.

WHO SHOULD DO FACIAL EXERCISES?

Your mirror will tell you if you need to do facial exercises. If the skin of your face appears softer and looser than it did a few years ago, if your nose, eyes, and chin seem to be losing their characteristic shapes, it is time to begin the exercises. The sooner you attack the aging process of the face with exercise, the easier it will be to achieve positive results. Generally, I recommend beginning exercises somewhere between thirty-five and forty.

Age, however, does not come all at once to the face. Your eyes may get smaller long before the flesh under the jawline stretches and sags, or vice versa. Many people destroy the elastic skin tone of their faces at an early age with crash diets (see chapter 5). If you are thirty-five and see one part of your face that conspicuously needs exercise, do the exercise intended to improve that part of the face only.

Facial exercises are definitely not for the smooth-skinned, youthful face. Although young people use no more facial muscles than their elders, nature ensures them a facial skin that is smooth and taut. The same is true of the body. A young woman may maintain her figure with little exercise, but as she ages, muscle cells deteriorate of their own accord, and if she doesn't begin to exercise, her lovely shape will disappear. Muscle cells refuse to rejuvenate themselves easily as you age, and you must accomplish what the body once did automatically with conscientious work. As the time comes for your body to slow down, you must speed up your efforts if you want to retard the aging process. Like Alice in Wonderland, you must run to stay in the same place.

PROVIDE THE RIGHT ATMOSPHERE

When you are ready to begin, you must provide an atmosphere that will encourage you to learn the facial exercises properly and enjoy doing them. It is especially important to maintain this atmosphere during your training period; once you really know the exercises you can do them anywhere—in the movies, in the bath, or while waiting for an elevator.

First, set aside a half hour of leisure time. Suspend all activities, all thoughts of pressing obligations. Pretend you are on an airplane, incommunicado, physically removed from everyday demands. No phone calls, no quick glances in the fridge to see if you have milk, no laundry. Forget worries as much as possible and attend to the moment.

Choose a quiet, pleasant spot in your home. Sit in front of a large mirror or bring a hand mirror with you. It is preferable to sit cross-legged, with a straight back, on the floor, but if you find this position uncomfortable, use a table and chair. Place this book and the mirror in front of you. Locate the facial atlas in the book (page 56) and mark the page so you can consult it easily. Prepare yourself to concentrate your full energies on the task at hand. Take the exercises seriously, even if you secretly consider them frivolous. I've noticed that most people will spend any amount of cash on things they consider self-indulgent, but they are reluctant to spend time. Remember, practicing exercises of any kind is a positive expression of genuine self-love.

Before you begin the exercises you must relax your face. Whenever you tense any part of the body, it is more difficult to move it freely. A tense neck, for example, cannot move as far to the right or left as a relaxed neck. With a relaxed face, you will find it easier to locate the muscles the facial exercises require you to move and also easier to move them.

Learning to relax the face is, in itself, a beautifying art. A tense face is usually a forbidding, unfriendly face. Tensions deepen facial lines and create an anxious, unpleasant expression. A tense face looks older, too. You will find that once you learn to relax your face at will, other people will be more open to you and more comfortable in your presence. Relaxing your face should become as much part of your preparation for a social occasion as applying makeup or combing your hair.

Cream your face

Use your favorite cream of the moment. It is not necessary to choose an especially rich or expensive cream, just one with a pleasant scent and texture that you enjoy. Place small dabs on your face and neck and massage gently with long, light strokes. Stroke from the center of

Facial Exercises
51

your face out toward the sides. Use both hands and gently cover your entire face and neck. The cream, combined with the massage, will lubricate your face, softening the skin and the muscles, and make you able to move it freely.

Locate the tense areas in your face

Before you can relax your face, you must become conscious of the tension there. Where does your face feel stiff, wooden, and tight? Is there a tense, pressured sensation in your jawbones, your forehead, or the back of your neck? Are your teeth clenched? Do your eyes feel swollen, dry, or irritated? Is it difficult to open and close them? Do your lips feel pinched? Feel your face with your hands. Look in the mirror. Is your forehead blank or furrowed with worry? Are there deep wrinkles along the sides of your nose? Are your lips narrow, pale, and stringy, or are they wide, large, content, and at rest?

Once you have located the tense areas, concentrate on them. If your forehead is tense, focus on it. Focus on your clenched teeth or tight lips. What are these tense areas telling you about your emotions? Often our inner feelings get swept away from our conscious minds in the flurry of daily activity and register only in our muscles. When you concentrate on the physical manifestations of tension—tight, unyielding muscles—and relax them, the source of tension may dissipate as well.

Breathe into your face

Now, relax your cheeks and let them hang. Pretend that your breath is a big wind that you are sending into your face to blow the tension away. Imagine your breath blowing into the tense areas. Feel those areas expand as the breath goes into them and relax as the breath leaves. This yogic exercise is primarily a psychic experience, since you can't actually send breath into your face. Psychic or not, it works. After five minutes of breathing into your face, you will feel your face and your entire body relax.

Relax your neck

Much of the tension in our facial expressions is the result of accumulated tension in the neck—one of the primary places the body stores tense and anxious feelings. Let your neck hang, and feel your head as if it were a heavy weight dangling on the end of your neck. Then slowly revolve your head in a circle—to the left, to the back, to the right, and to the front again. This exercise should help release the tension in both your face and neck.

GET ACQUAINTED WITH THE MUSCLES OF
YOUR FACE

Once your face is relaxed, it is time to learn where the facial muscles are located and how they move. This will help you accomplish the subtle movements required by the exercises. Begin by studying the facial atlas on page 56. Then pass both hands over your face and neck, touching and exploring every part. Compare the muscles noted on the atlas to the structures you feel with your hands.

Facial Exercises

Isolation exercises

These are exercises in which you isolate one muscle from those surrounding it and move only one part of your face at a time. Many of my exercises require you to isolate and move only one set of facial muscles. These warm-ups are good practice.

Move only one eyebrow.
Move one cheek.
Try to move one of your ears.
Move the right side of your mouth, then the left.

Consult the mirror to make certain you are moving only one part of your face at a time. This may be more difficult than it sounds, and it will take some practice to get the hang of it.

Pull your nose down toward your upper lip. Note that you are not using the muscles in your nose but the muscles in your upper lip to do this. Feel how the upper lip connects with the nose. Now try to move your nose without moving your lips as well.

Squinching the face

Squeeze your face together tightly, as if you were trying to make your eyes, nose, chin, and cheeks meet at a point in the center of your face. Feel the tip of your chin, your lips, and your forehead. Squinch, hold, and let go. Try again. Notice that the muscles you are using to perform this exercise are located in a circle near the center of your face and that you are not using any of the muscles around your cheeks or hairline. Your face is tightened because the muscles around the mouth are pulling forward, while the muscles on the sides of your face go

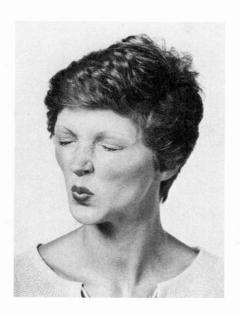

along with the motion. This exercise will activate the muscles of your face and at the same time help you to become conscious of the specific function of a muscle.

THE FACIAL EXERCISES

Now you are ready to learn the exercises. Read the instructions for each exercise from beginning to end before you try it. As you perform an exercise, observe your face carefully in the mirror and compare your expression at the completed phase with the expression on the face in the illustration. Make sure you are not committing any of the "Don'ts"—some are also shown—which are common mistakes, easy to make when you first learn an exercise. It helps to visualize in your mind's eye your own face performing the same movement you see in the illustration.

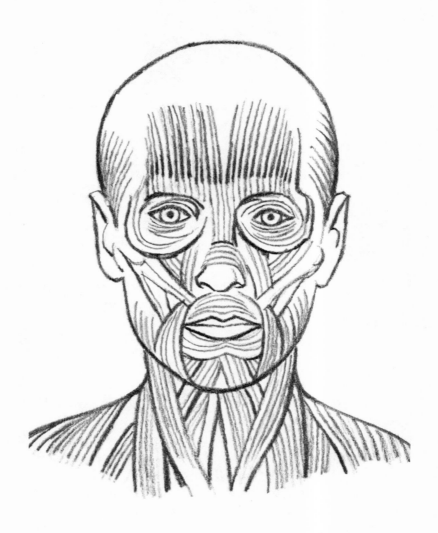

Facelift Without Surgery
56

You will notice that there are only nine basic exercises, designed to strengthen the muscles in the jaws, the lips, the eyes, the cheeks, and the nose and to tighten the loose skin on the neck below the jaw. Once you have mastered the basic exercises and feel comfortable with them, you may want to learn the supplementary exercises which follow them. The more exercises you do, of course, the better the results will be. It is more important, however, to do fewer exercises regularly and properly than to do many in a haphazard, inconsistent fashion.

The movements that the exercises require are subtle, and because they involve using muscles you haven't used before, you should expect to encounter some difficulty at first. Don't be disappointed if an exercise does not seem vigorous or dramatic; the exercises are based on isometric principles (pulling and pushing muscles) and are actually quite strenuous. You can expect to feel a slight ache in your facial muscles if you perform them properly. After the entire range of exercises is finished, your face should feel pleasantly invigorated, with a noticeable tingling sensation in the muscles.

If the exercises make you feel tense at first, get up and stretch your arms into the air, then bend down and touch your toes with your fingertips. Let your head hang down, and move it from side to side. Breathe deeply in and out. As you exhale, you will feel your body drop farther down toward your toes. Finally, straighten up slowly, vertebra by vertebra, until your head is in a straight line with your neck and spine. Do this between each exercise or whenever you feel tense.

Exercise 1. The cheeks

WHAT IT DOES: Though we use some of the muscles in our cheeks to smile, we rarely use the cheek muscles lying just in front of the ears, which tend to grow soft and slack with age. Exercise 1 tightens sagging cheek muscles so they become firmer and more taut.

HOW TO PERFORM: Open your eyes. Clench your teeth gently and grin as hard as possible. Usually, you use the muscles in the part of your cheeks closest to your mouth to grin. For this exercise try to reach back to your ears with your grin and then to your hairline. When you do this, you allow the muscles in front of your ears to do the work. Visualize the grin reaching back to your ears. Hold the expression for ten seconds and let go. Repeat ten times. After ten repetitions you will feel the muscles near your hairline and in front of your ears reverberating. You will also feel blood rushing into your cheeks.

DON'TS: Don't use the muscles around your mouth; use the muscles near your ears to pull your lips back into the grin. If you experiment and try using both sets of muscles to create the same expression, you will see that there is a distinct difference in the way the exercise looks and feels when you use the muscles near your ears.

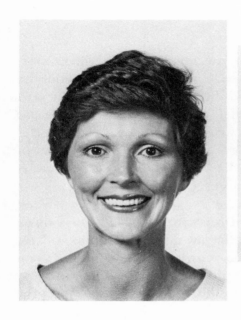
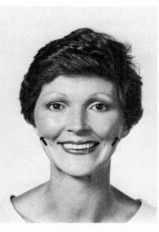

Exercise 2. The jaw muscles

WHAT IT DOES: The jaw muscles and the cheek muscles are connected. As we age the muscles that fill out the cheeks begin to sink, and the muscles just above the jaws become looser and heavier. Despite the fact that we use our jaws to eat and talk, we do not employ all the muscles in the jaw area. Exercise 2 puts seldom-used muscles of the jaws, cheeks, and neck to work and makes the muscles that fill out the cheeks larger and firmer.

HOW TO PERFORM: Drop your lower jaw as far down as it will go. Don't force the jaw downward; relax it. Now hook three fingers behind your lower teeth and use them to push the jaw farther down. With the fingers firmly planted over the teeth, push the lower jaw up to meet the upper jaw. Your fingers will act as a weight, making you use more muscles, more forcefully, to move your jaw upward. Close your jaws slowly. You can feel all the muscles operating in your jaws, cheeks, and neck with your hand. Repeat three times, then relax the face.

DON'TS: Don't stick out your neck; keep it in a vertical line with your spine. When you extend your neck, you unconsciously use neck muscles to help jaw muscles do the work, which makes the exercise less effective.

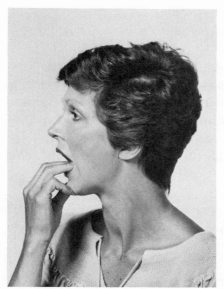 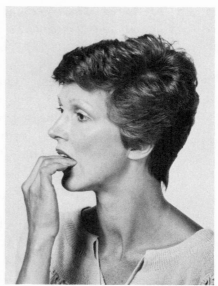

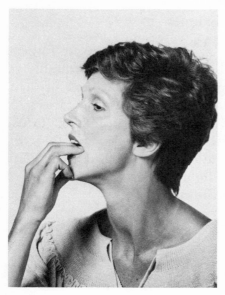

DON'T

*Exercise 3. The corners of the mouth, the area
surrounding the mouth, and the skin on the lower
jawline*

WHAT IT DOES: The skin of the lower jaw often sags
earlier than other parts of the face. This exercise tightens
the skin on the lower jaw and helps preserve its contours.
At the same time, it smooths the skin surrounding the
mouth and prevents the corners of the mouth from
drooping.

HOW TO PERFORM: Place all four fingers of both
hands gently on your cheeks at the point where the jaw
muscles end. Pucker your lips and use the muscles of
your cheeks, which extend down to the lower jaw, to pull
your face forward. Visualize your cheeks and jaw muscles
pulling your face forward. Your fingers hold back the
flesh of your cheeks, forcing your cheek and jaw muscles
to work harder. Repeat six times.

DON'TS: Don't pull on the face with your fingers.
Facial skin should never be pulled or handled roughly, or
it may stretch. As you pucker your lips, think of them
moving in a forward direction, not just any old way. If
your lips move forward, it will be easier for you to use
your cheek and jaw muscles to pull your face forward,
too. In other words, all the muscles you use in your face
to perform this exercise should be moving in a forward
direction. Don't stick out the chin.

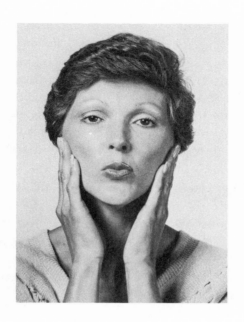

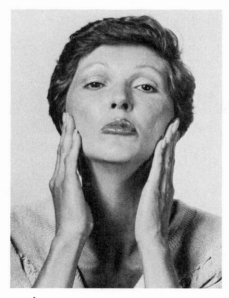

DON'T

Exercise 4. The mouth

WHAT IT DOES: With age the area around the mouth puckers, giving the lips a pinched, disapproving expression. Exercise 4 animates and strengthens the muscle tissue around the mouth. Although this exercise cannot remove wrinkles, it makes the mouth area appear fuller and helps smooth wrinkles out.

HOW TO PERFORM: Make a light pout with the lips so that they come to a point. Now, press the area around your mouth into your teeth using the muscles around your mouth. Think of the area around your mouth as a complete circle, and concentrate on making sure that every part of this circle presses inward and touches the teeth. Remember, you are pressing your lips not into your teeth (they are pouting) but into the area *around* your mouth. Press and hold for ten seconds. Repeat three times. Your face will feel tense after this exercise; to relax, move it, blow through your cheeks, and let your cheeks hang.

DON'TS: With this exercise there is a tendency to tense the nose and back of the neck and thus to involve these areas. This is the wrong approach. Use only the muscles around the mouth. The pout you make with your lips should be gentle; don't squinch and squeeze your mouth.

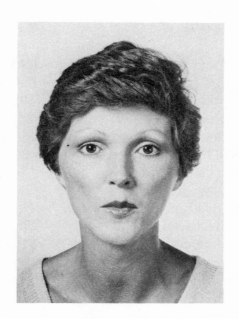

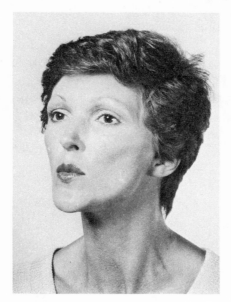

DON'T

Exercise 5. The forehead

WHAT IT DOES: There are few muscles in the upper
and middle part of the forehead, and we do little to exercise the ones that are there. With age the flesh under the
skin of the forehead becomes skimpy and blood circulation is impeded. This exercise tones and smooths the
forehead by filling out the muscles beneath its skin and
improving circulation in the area.

HOW TO PERFORM: Take both index fingers and
place them directly under the eyebrows. The tips of your
fingers should be resting at the root of your nose. Then,
using only the muscles above the eyes, press your forehead down while you keep your fingers in the same place.
Visualize your forehead attempting to push your fingers
out of place. Close your eyes while you perform the exercise. Repeat six times. Afterward wriggle your nose and
face like a rabbit to relax.

DON'TS: Don't stick your neck out or lean elbows on
a table. Don't push your fingers up. Relax your fingers
and let your forehead do the work of pushing downward.

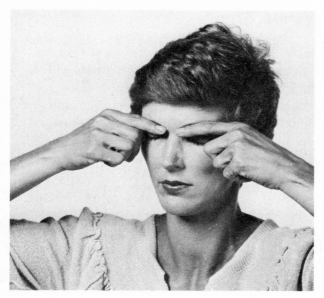

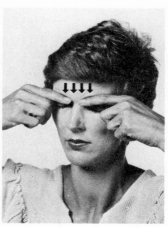

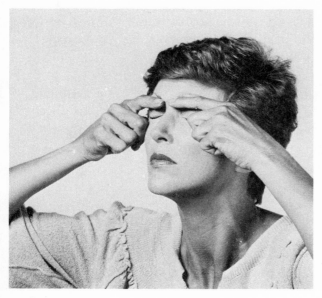

DON'T

Exercise 6. The eye

WHAT IT DOES: With age the eyes tend to shrink in size because the ring of muscles which keeps them wide and open gets smaller and weaker. Exercise 6 helps to enlarge the eye by strengthening the powerful muscles surrounding it. The exercise may also reduce puffiness beneath the eye by increasing the circulation in the area, which will help disperse accumulated liquids and fats.

HOW TO PERFORM: Look straight ahead and keep the eyes as wide open as possible, without actually forcing them open or using any muscles but the eye muscles. Relax the eye in its open position and slowly and deliberately bring the lower lid up to meet the upper lid. It helps to visualize the lower lid rising to meet the upper lid. Hold the position to the count of ten, then relax. Repeat six times. This exercise brings into play the muscle in the lower eyelid, which we do not normally use to open and close the eye. Afterward, close your eyes, let your cheeks hang, and relax the whole face.

DON'TS: Don't move the upper eyelid, or squinch eyes, forehead, or any other part of the face. The face should remain relaxed and only the lower eyelid should move. Don't look up, but stare straight ahead.

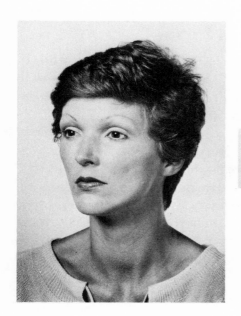

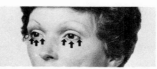

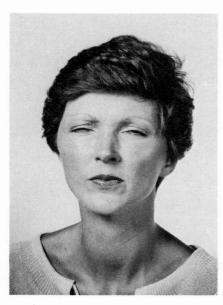

DON'T

Exercise 7. The chin

WHAT IT DOES: The flesh beneath the chin tends to become skimpy with age. The skin gives and appears to hang loosely. Exercise 7 firms up the two large muscles that create the buttressing structure of the chin.

HOW TO PERFORM: Relax the face and keep it as serene as possible. Consult the atlas and note the two large, round muscles that form the chin. Then concentrate and pull these muscles away from each other. Move the muscle on the right to the right and the muscle on the left to the left. You are actually using the two muscles to pull them apart. This sounds mysterious but is quite easy to perform, though when you look in the mirror you will not see much visible action. You will be able to feel the muscles in the chin pulling in opposite directions. Keep your eyes closed to help you concentrate. Repeat ten times.

DON'TS: Don't tense the back of your neck or stick out your chin. Keep your chin relaxed. Involve your lower lip as little as possible.

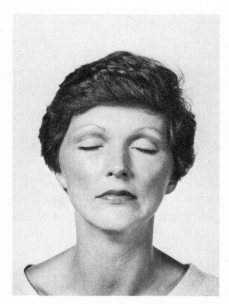
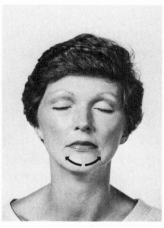

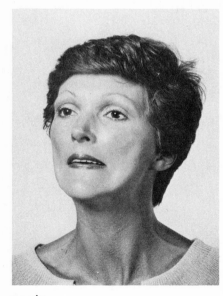

DON'T

Exercise 8. The area beneath the chin and the jaw

WHAT IT DOES: This exercise tightens the skin beneath the chin and jaw, which stretches and sags with age, causing the lower part of the face to lose its youthful contour.

HOW TO PERFORM: Cross your hands over your chest. Stick out your chin, as in the first photograph. You will feel the skin under your jaw tighten immediately when you do this. Turn your chin slowly to the right and then to the left, keeping it extended. Repeat ten times. The skin beneath the jaw pulls and tightens as you move your chin.

DON'TS: Don't tense the neck. Relax all your muscles except the muscles beneath the jaw and chin. Don't bend your chin down toward your shoulders or raise it toward the ceiling. Keep it at shoulder level.

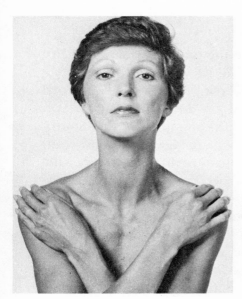
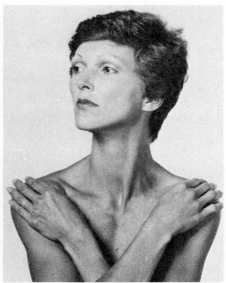

Exercise 9. The nose

WHAT IT DOES: Because the muscles which hold up the nose weaken with age, the tip of the nose tends to droop and hang forward. Gravity increases this misfortune by pulling the loosened tip down. The tip of the nose itself has no muscles, but the muscles in the mouth area, beneath the nose and at the bridge of the nose, can be strengthened to help pull the nose back up again. The exercise also firms the area above the upper lip.

HOW TO PERFORM: Pretend you are a rabbit and push your upper lip up and down three times rapidly. Then, pull your mouth and upper lip down and hold them in that position. Repeat the sequence ten times. Visualize the muscles in your mouth pulling the nose down.

DON'TS: Don't involve your cheeks in the exercise. Keep the lips even; don't extend your upper lip over your lower lip. Don't use the lip muscles to lift your lip, but use the muscles at the saddle (or middle area) of your nose.

SUPPLEMENTARY EXERCISES

Once you have mastered these nine basic exercises, you may want to add the following five supplementary exercises to your repertoire. These exercises will improve the muscle tone of the face in different areas, or in different ways, from the basic exercises.

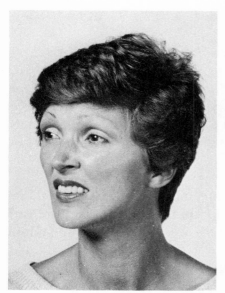 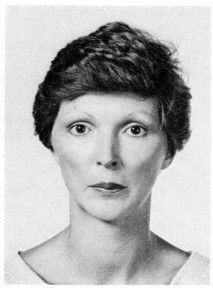

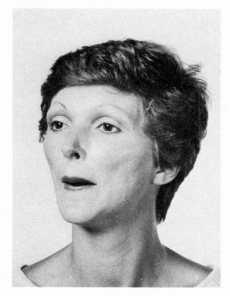

DON'T

Supplementary exercise 1. The area below the jaw

WHAT IT DOES: Firms up the skin below the jaw.

HOW TO PERFORM: Stick out your chin and push the underside of your right jaw muscles toward your chin. Slowly turn your face to the left, hold, and turn back to the center. Then do the same thing on the other side. Do three times to each side.

DON'TS: Don't use your mouth to push the flesh beneath your jaw toward your chin. Relax the mouth. Don't turn your head too far to the side because you will strain the muscles of your neck.

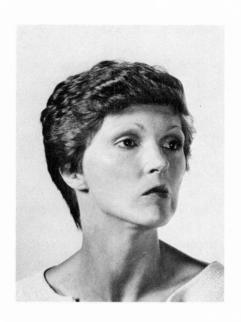

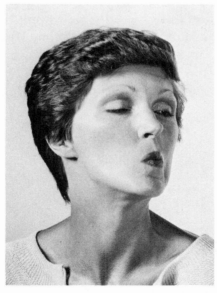

DON'T

Supplementary exercise 2. The mouth

WHAT IT DOES: Firms up the corners of the mouth to help prevent them from drooping.

HOW TO PERFORM: Pout lips slightly. Concentrate on the right corner of the mouth and very slowly press it into your teeth. Use the muscles at the corner of your mouth to perform the "pressing" action. Push the right corner of the mouth along the teeth to the center of the mouth. Then change sides and do the same exercise on the left. It should take ten seconds for the corner of your mouth to reach the center of your mouth. You may find it difficult to change sides at first because you will be totally focused on only one side of your mouth. Do three times to each side.

DON'TS: If you are working with the right side of your mouth, don't use the left side to pull the lips to the center. The pushing action should come from the right corner of the mouth. The exercise only works if the opposite side of the mouth does not pull. The same thing, of course, is true when you do the exercise on the left side.

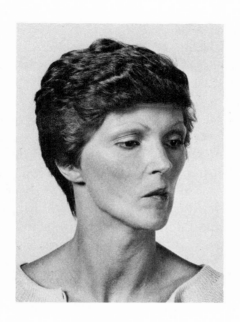

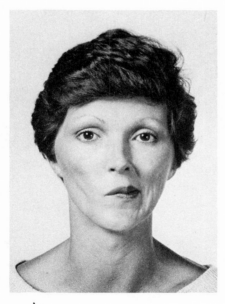

DON'T

Supplementary exercise 3. The nose

WHAT IT DOES: Firms up the muscles which keep the nose from drooping.

HOW TO PERFORM: Locate the muscle at the root of the nose, between the eyes and under the forehead, on your atlas. You must see and understand the location of that muscle before you begin to use it. Keep your face immobile and concentrate on the spot between the eyebrows. Now, try to pull the eyebrows up and pull the muscle *in,* toward the back of your head, at the same time. This exercise is impossible to illustrate with a photograph (although the model in our photograph is performing it) because it takes place below the level of the skin.

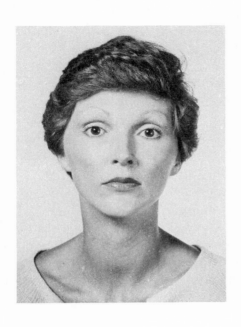

Supplementary exercise 4. The area between the upper lip and the nose

WHAT IT DOES: Firms up the area between the nose and upper lip and makes it smoother.

HOW TO PERFORM: Open mouth slightly and pull your upper lip down over your upper teeth to the lower lip. Imagine your upper lip rolling down over your teeth as if it were a window shade.

DON'TS: Don't use your nose or cheeks. Keep your entire face relaxed. Be sure to isolate the area between your nose and upper lip, and move it gently. Don't grin to get your upper lip down; relax your mouth.

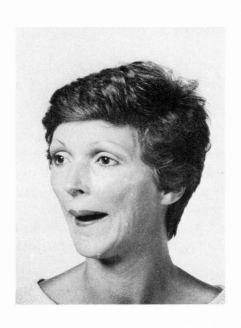

Supplementary exercise 5. The eyes

WHAT IT DOES: Revitalizes and relaxes the eye area.
Keeps nerves and capillaries in the eye area in good
shape.

HOW TO PERFORM: Eye rolls are an old-fashioned
but very important exercise for the face. Roll the eyes in a
clockwise direction, first looking up, then to the side, then
down, then to the other side, then up again. Try to see
objects on all points of the imaginary clock and to extend
your vision as far as possible. Do three times in a clockwise direction, then three times counterclockwise.

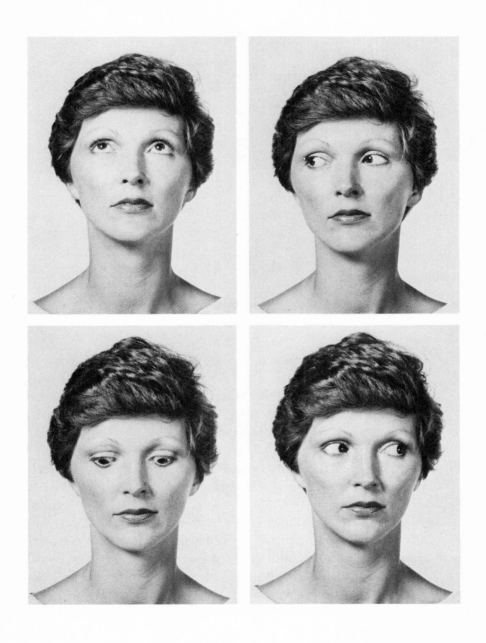

4 *Body Exercises*

Doctors and gerontologists are telling us with increasing urgency that regular exercise is essential for a long and healthy life. This advice is based on more than mere conjecture. Studies have proved that those who engage in regular, strenuous exercise are far less susceptible to cardiovascular disease than those who don't. Why? Muscles throughout the body enlarge and increase in power with repeated exercise—including that all-important muscle, the heart.

As the muscle fibers which make up the heart become stronger through exercise, they are able to contract with more force and send an increased volume of blood and oxygen to working muscles. As a result, the well-exercised heart does its work more efficiently and develops greater immunity to strain. Exercise, moreover, keeps the blood flowing freely through the heart, dislodging sediments which settle in the coronary arteries and valves. If these sediments accumulate, they impair the function of the heart and block the flow of blood and oxygen to the body.

Because exercise improves circulation, it helps the body to rid itself of wastes faster, and it causes blood vessels in the muscles and skin to dilate, which reduces blood pressure and improves the ability of the blood to dissolve clots. Exercise increases the rate and depth of breathing, so respiratory muscles, too, are strengthened. And because the bones and skeletal muscles remain strong only if they are used, and otherwise become fragile with age, exercise is an excellent insurance policy for the skeleton. In short, those who would stay healthy must heed the old Chinese saying, "If you don't trouble your body, it will trouble you."

WHAT EXERCISE DOES FOR YOUR FACE

Possibly because we are unable to see our hearts, blood vessels, and bones or notice the dire effect of lack of exercise on our internal organs until we are actually sick, these arguments do little to persuade the sedentary among us to jog, play tennis, or enroll in a gymnastics class. We can, however, see the outsides of our bodies, which are just as severely affected by lack of exercise as our internal selves.

Many of the unattractive body formations we dismiss as the inevitable result of the aging process are more likely the results of lack of exercise. Although we think of a flabby body afflicted with a potbelly, sagging buttocks, dimpled thighs, and hanging upper arms as the mandatory physique of middle age, the same flabby body can

Body Exercises
87

belong to anyone, at any age, who refuses to exercise. When we are twenty, however, natural processes cooperate by working in our favor instead of doing their best to destroy the figure as they do later on.

As we pass the middle years, we can expect even less attractive and more decrepit images to greet us in the mirror unless we exercise. The perversely sedentary suffer from wrinkled skin across the chest and dowager's humps, or rounded upper backs. As muscles grow weaker, the posture becomes worse, and the entire body more fragile and less vigorous. Aches, kinks, and weakened muscles affect the way we look as well as how we feel.

Those who do not exercise stand, walk, and move poorly—they navigate with a listless plod. With good reason, they begin to question their ability to accomplish unfamiliar movements or even necessary tasks. The unexercised are apt to suffer from freak accidents—such as bending down to pick a flower and putting their back out for a week. If you think these crippling and unattractive syndromes are the automatic accompaniments of old age, take a good look at any older person you know who has always exercised religiously. There is a sixty-five-year-old man in my yoga class who has the basic silhouette and muscle tone of a young man, and my lithe and youthful mother—in her late seventies—not only does vigorous gymnastics but teaches them seven days a week!

It seems reasonable that exercise should improve the health and physique, you may say, but how does exercise affect the face? The increased blood circulation resulting from exercise nourishes the facial skin with a supply of oxygen and removes impurities. With exercise the color brightens, the eyes sparkle, and the skin becomes softer and smoother. Exercise, too, reduces tension in the neck and upper back. Unreleased, this tension makes the face look drawn and pinched and may lead to groggy feelings and headaches. I can always tell when a friend doesn't exercise. Her skin is cloudy, her eyes are dull, and her color is sallow or ashen. If she smokes and maintains late hours, these negative aspects are magnified. To me, no amount of makeup or artificial lighting can disguise this dull, listless, tense quality in a face. It is more unattractive than any wrinkle or imperfect feature I can imagine.

THE PSYCHIC BENEFITS OF EXERCISE

The psychic benefits of exercise are not often emphasized by the medical profession or beauty experts. However, people who exercise proclaim that exercise makes them feel good, mentally as well as physically, and that it is guaranteed to raise the spirits when they are low. Why? So far science has given us no reason why this should be true.

I believe that every human being has an instinctive need for movement. A healthy child is full of energy, moving, running, and jumping all the time. However, when children are old enough to go to school they are forced to sit still at their desks. They learn that it is not polite to fidget, jump up and down, or move around too vigorously in houses, buses, and theaters. They learn to sublimate their need for movement and sit still. This repressed energy, I believe, is converted into psychic tension—particularly in city dwellers, whose stress level is greater and whose opportunities to move around are less.

The less we move the more phlegmatic, restless, and anxious we feel. If we have never exercised regularly, we may not even realize how tense or anxious we feel or be aware that we are sublimating our need for movement. Our bodies are comfortably inert, and we attribute these unpleasant feelings to some other cause. This is not to deny that there are many reasons, often good ones, to feel negative emotions. I am convinced, however, that exercise offers us an inimitable outlet for anger, aggression, and anxiety, while lack of exercise augments these emotions, bottles them in, and allows them to settle into our muscles and stay there, taking the form of lethargy and depression. Needless to say, these negative emotions are also reflected in the face.

Anyone who plays tennis knows the liberating feeling smashing a ball across the court can give, especially if you feel angry. Joggers experience the relaxed, free sensation of a five-mile run. As soon as my friends begin an exercise program, they invariably comment, "I feel so good." Perhaps because exercise forces you to concentrate on an activity that has nothing to do with the endless machinations of the mind, you inevitably feel released and more content afterward. This feeling of release may be temporary, but it is better than no release at all or one obtained by damaging your health with tranquilizers and alcohol.

Those who exercise always have greater confidence, a feeling of security about the body, and a sense of its grace and power that is reflected in their total bearing and the attitude they communicate to others. People involved in physical activities radiate an energetic sensuality, an aura that draws others to them like a magnet. If you have friends who jog, swim, or play a sport religiously, you will notice a confident vitality to their movements. Like healthy animals, they are sensuous, relaxed, and filled with energy. Whatever their age, they seem younger. They walk better, run better, sleep better, wear clothes better, feel better, and look better than people who never move.

If you have practiced some form of exercise all your life, the preceding information will not be news to you. Fortunately, more and more people are getting the message that exercise makes them look and feel better and is essential for good health. In Central Park I see people jogging and playing basketball at all hours of the night. The New York health clubs and Ys are overbooked for the first time in history. Women I know are engaging in physical activities that most women have never done before—like lifting weights and studying the martial arts. But despite the many people who are making sports and movement an integral part of their lives, there are still too many who do not exercise. Why not?

For a long time physical fitness was considered neither necessary nor chic in the United States. When we came to New York from Germany, I was astonished to see how little emphasis the American public placed on exercise. Whereas in Europe, the majority of people did gymnastics, participated in sports, and rode bicycles as a means of transportation, here people seemed to enjoy watching sports more than doing them and drove their cars whenever possible. My mother, who taught gymnastics, had only a few students enrolled in her classes when she first began teaching here, and most of those were Europeans. Exercising with any degree of enthusiasm was considered anti-intellectual. Even today, most colleges require only one physical education credit for graduation. If you are part of the no-exercise generation, it may be especially difficult for you to convince yourself it's time to enter the physical fitness age.

Actually, it's not easy for anyone to exercise regularly. Our bodies do not know what is good for them and are comfortable in a state of lassitude, and this is difficult to overcome. Even those of us who love to exercise can always think of a hundred good reasons not to do so when the moment arrives to pull ourselves out of bed and begin jogging on a drizzly morning, to betake ourselves to the swimming pool on a cold day, or to attend an evening dance class after a hard day of work. Although I have exercised all my life and cannot imagine life without exercise, when I return from a vacation I do not rush back to my dance classes; I procrastinate. My body, in those few weeks, has lost its addiction to exercise, and I have once again become inert.

For those who have never exercised or who have done so only sporadically, it is a heroic task to begin. Until the body becomes accustomed to exercise and learns to rejoice in its pleasures, exercise for most of us is simply an unpleasant form of work that is displacing something we would much rather do—like going to the movies. Moreover, when we first begin to exercise after a long period of inertia, our bodies ache; we feel inept and embarrassed as our lack of coordination and muscle power become painfully apparent. We may feel a bit better afterward, but the moment a greater attraction or more pressing responsibility intrudes, we cancel our commitment to exercise. "I'd love to take that gymnastics class," we moan, "but I simply haven't the time," or "That pool is so dirty, and what will I do with my hair afterward," or "I hate getting dressed and undressed, and I'll be bushed when I finish," or "I'm expecting someone for dinner, and I really have to clean the house." These are all good excuses and, at the same time, irrelevant. It always amazes me that people consider almost *anything* more important and more convenient than exercise. Why should an activity which is so good for us and ultimately so pleasurable be so hard to do?

The reason, I believe, is that exercise is the only function you perform exclusively for your own benefit. There is no audience to cheer you on or to praise you, there is no monetary reward, and there is no one else who derives the slightest benefit from it. Exercise is only for you, for your health and your enjoyment. When you are exercising you are totally involved in your own body, and in this Puritan society that is somehow an unchristian form of work. You will always make time to do other jobs—to go to school, to clean, to help others, or to work overtime at the office—for these activities are virtuous. Exercise, on the other hand, is a narcissistic activity—it gives nothing to anyone but you. Trying on fifty sweaters at a department store or spending three hours at a beauty salon are also narcissistic activities, but they involve no pain or labor, and for this reason you like to do them. Exercise, despite the benefits or pleasures you derive from it, is first and foremost *work*. There is no way around that.

WHAT TO EXPECT FROM EXERCISE

When people first begin to exercise, they often feel disappointed. Because they have heard so much about the value of exercise, they expect an immediate change in their lives—the way they feel and look. Unfortunately, no one thing can drastically alter your whole life. Exercise will improve your health, appearance, and vitality but only after you have put in many hours of effort. I have often seen friends begin to jog, play a sport, or study dance and rave that they feel marvelous, transformed. Inevitably, these people drop out soon after they begin. The results they feel at first are largely preconditioned responses, and they do not realize how much discipline their exercise will require of them, or the complexities involved.

Whatever form of exercise you choose, doing it will put you through many ups and downs—physically and emotionally—if you stick with it. At first you will feel elated, high, energized. However, you will also experience self-consciousness and frustration because you are unable to run or swim as long as you want or to perform movements and strokes which look so simple when someone else does them. Over a period of time, you will feel your power accumulating, your expertise growing; you will become conscious of the way many muscles work and become able to use them more efficiently. You will learn to release muscles at will, then contract them to perform various functions. You will gradually attain skills you never before possessed.

Expertise comes at a different rate for everyone. In this process there are constant setbacks; one day you will feel elated because you performed a feat you could not do the day before, and the next day you will feel tired, weak, and inept again. Remember, talent and coordination are only small parts of learning an exercise or sport; the rest, quite literally, is perspiration. Think how many thousands of times a professional tennis player hits the ball to perfect a particular stroke or how many laps an Olympic swimmer does every day. It often takes years to master the skills of the exercise you practice regularly—

years before you can jog five miles, smash a tennis ball across the net, or get your head to your knees in exercise class. However, as you accept the challenge, become more involved in the subtleties your muscles have to offer, and watch your power and proficiency increase, you will become more and more addicted to your chosen exercise. By "addicted" I mean that you will feel lousy when you don't exercise and good when you do.

DON'T KID YOURSELF

I have many friends who complain that they exercise regularly yet notice no change in the way they look or feel. People often fool themselves; they think they are exercising when actually they are not.

There is a man at the gym I attend who lies flat on his back on the slant board for at least ten minutes. I am sure he is convinced that he does sit-ups. Some women I know spend an hour chatting at the poolside and tell me they swim every day. There are ski enthusiasts who recline with a hot grog by the lodge fireplace, dressed to kill in fashionable ski outfits. Exercise means *doing* it, not merely partaking of the proper atmosphere. Even in gymnastics, yoga, or dance classes, there are two ways to participate in the movements: with minimum energy or with maximum vitality and body force. You can barely raise your arm in a lethargic stretch, or you can vigorously raise the same arm. Needless to say, it is the latter technique that improves your health and appearance. Exercise must be electric—full of energy—to be truly beneficial.

I have often heard friends say, "I don't really need to join a formal exercise class. I get plenty of exercise just walking to my job and doing my housework." Many people believe that they are exercising when they scrub the floor, climb a flight of stairs, or walk to work. They are moving, but they are not exercising.

There are many aspects to exercise. First, real exercise is a formal ritual which asks you to use and develop your muscles in a specific fashion for specific ends. Housework does not say, "Raise that arm in a particular way and do thus and so with it"; it says, "Get the floor clean." In fact, because housework is basically boring and tiring, we would rather use as few muscles as possible to do it.

Formal exercise, on the other hand, is enjoyable; you watch the sun shine over a clear lake as you swim; you take in the early morning, the bedewed grass of the park as you jog; you admire the white mountain as you ski. Even if you exercise in an urban environment, there is the enjoyment of accomplishment, of watching your body become more beautiful and powerful. You wash the floor or hang up the laundry not in order to improve your strength or appearance or to develop a skill but to get the floor clean or the laundry dry. The movements you make are not for you; there is nothing narcissistic about them. As for walking and climbing stairs, these activities are more healthful than driving or taking an elevator, but they are not really formal exercise.

Another reason people fail to experience the benefits of exercise is that they do not exercise often enough. The best way to maintain your health and youthful physique is to exercise almost every day. I personally believe that two exercise sessions—one in the morning and one in the afternoon or night—are necessary to stave off the aging process effectively; but few people are as fanatic on the subject of exercise as I. A minimum of three sessions a week, however, is the least amount of time you can spend exercising and derive real results.

Experts tell us that muscles in the body which are contracted during exercise relax back to their original state of tension after only thirty-six hours. So, if you jump rope or attend a modern dance class once a week, you may enjoy yourself, slightly increase your stamina and skill, and feel better afterward, but you are doing relatively little to improve your health and physique. "Three times a week!" you may moan, thinking you deserve the medal of honor for having gotten yourself to the exercise class, tennis court, or swimming pool at least once. The truth may be hard to hear, but if you really want to look and feel younger, you have to face it. Remember, once you become addicted to exercise, three sessions a week will seem as crucial to your well-being as eating dinner.

THE KINDS OF EXERCISE YOU NEED

In my opinion, two types of exercise are necessary to maintain health and vitality: a strenuous or aerobic-type exercise, which strengthens the cardiovascular system and develops endurance and stamina, and a calisthenic exercise, which stretches and tones the muscles, makes the body firm and relaxes it, and removes the lumps and bulges caused by accumulations of fat. Calisthenic exercises also prepare the muscles for sports, which may cause injuries if you aren't in shape. Exercises classified as strenuous are jogging, swimming, jumping rope, handball, squash, or a vigorous game of tennis. Exercises which are not strenuous are golf, volleyball, any ball game that you are just learning to play (and spending a lot of time chasing the ball or standing around while your partner chases it), bicycling on flat ground, and walking. Swimming is only strenuous if you swim with energy and vitality. When a strenuous exercise is done properly, it should make you pant.

If you are out of shape and attempting an aerobic exercise for the first time in years, take it slowly. If your health is suspect, or if you are over thirty-five and have been sedentary most of your life, it is advisable to have a medical examination, including an electrocardiogram, before you begin. During intense exercise the muscles require more oxygen and place a greater demand on the heart to send it to them. If the heart is unaccustomed to pumping at an increased speed and is unable to keep pace with the body's need for oxygen, it may be damaged by its efforts. The muscles, too, may suffer from an oxygen deficit and accumulate lactic acid, which causes fatigue and impairs the function of the heart. At first, intersperse your jogging with walking, swim slowly, play a sport for a short period of time; do *not* push yourself to the point of exhaustion. I recommend consulting a book devoted to the exercise you want to practice before beginning.

Calisthenic exercises include Hatha Yoga (the Indian system for stretching and relaxing the muscles and stimulating the functions of the internal organs); modern, jazz, or ballet dancing (also strenuous); acrobatics; gymnastics; and any of the martial arts (which can also be strenuous). Tai Chi, a Chinese calisthenic which is becoming popular in this country, is especially recommended for older people or those who are recovering from an illness or are very out of shape. Its slow, graceful, gentle movements improve the flexibility, circulation, coordination, and balance in an unstrenuous fashion. The Japanese yoga called Makko-Ho consists of a few stretches which, by themselves, give maximum flexibility over a period of time.

If you have never exercised regularly or have begun many sports or exercises and then quit, making exercise an integral part of your weekly schedule will be difficult. Your body and mind will protest, and until you begin to feel the benefits of your exercise regime and see your new, improved body and enjoy it, you will literally have to force yourself to do it. You will dream up endless excuses not to go to your triweekly sessions and honestly believe they are legitimate preventive factors. If you are leading a busy, hectic life, it will be easy to find a vacant time slot for your exercise program. Some suggestions on how to fit exercise into your life follow.

Analyze your day for time slots

If you would like to exercise but cannot imagine when you will find time to do so, examine your day for an hour or two of unpressured time. Can you set your alarm a half hour or an hour earlier to make space for a morning session? You may find it convenient to attend an exercise class right after work, before you go home. Usually you would spend that hour "relaxing"—perusing the mail, watching the news on TV with a cocktail, or chatting on the telephone. Why not exercise instead? Exercise will provide your tense mind and muscles with a greater sense of relaxation than reclining on the sofa. If you work at home, you may be able to postpone your dinner preparations for an hour. Your gym or health club may have facilities for showering, enabling you to wash your hair and

Body Exercises
99

apply makeup there and save the time you would use for grooming at home. The weekend, of course, is an excellent time to exercise.

If you are on a pressured schedule, try to combine exercise with another activity or substitute it for one you already do. If you work, lunch hour is a good time to exercise. In an urban area there is undoubtedly a health club, YMCA, or dance studio near your job which holds classes or opens its facilities in the early afternoon. Many people like to jog during lunch hour. If you are overweight, this may be a good opportunity to skip an elaborate, sedentary lunch. Few people feel hungry after exercising. Later, you can grab some yogurt or a piece of fruit at your desk.

Combine exercise with social activities

Instead of inviting a friend to join you for dinner, invite him or her to join you for a gymnastics class or swim with dinner to follow. Suggest a basketball or tennis date to your husband, romantic interest, or friend. You may find it as enjoyable to spend an evening, either with a friend or alone, at a health club as at the movies. Seeing other people working out will inspire you, and you will meet new friends who share your interest.

Find an exercise you enjoy

Some types of exercise are simply not meant for some people. Although jogging is now a national fad, you may feel terrible before, during, and after you jog, though none of your friends would miss a day. Swimming in a chlorinated pool may destroy your sinuses and your hair and, even with protective goggles, irritate your eyes. You may feel so inept at tennis that learning is a trauma akin to birth.

You cannot be sure you despise any form of exercise, however, until you have given it a good two-month trial period with regular sessions. Naturally, the first few times you jog, dance, or swim, the unfamiliar experience will be difficult and possibly painful. You can expect to find yourself inept at any sport or gymnastics for several months, sometimes longer. Give the type of exercise you choose a chance before you renounce it. Unless the pain is sharp and crippling, it is merely your body's silent voice telling you, "I need this." Sometimes pains are the result of doing the exercise incorrectly. Don't wait until normal muscle pain completely vanishes, however, before you exercise again. If you do, you will negate the effects of your first, difficult session.

Before you attempt any exercise, ask yourself what attracts you to it. Are you going to jog because your husband does, or because there is something you find intrinsically appealing about jogging—moving through space with your feet rhythmically pounding the earth, for example. If jogging seems silly to you, and you hate leaving the house and putting on special clothes to do it, try jumping rope instead. The benefits are the same but the rhythm and skills demanded are different. Also, you can jump rope anywhere without special clothing or shoes.

I have often heard friends declare that *their* sport is skiing, jai alai, scuba diving, or some other activity impossible to do regularly in the area where they live. Your exercise should never be one you can only do once or twice a season or at great inconvenience or expense. Settle for one you can do easily, on a regular basis. Remember, nobody is too old, too inept, or too out of shape to do some form of exercise.

Get proper instruction

There is a right way to do any sport or exercise and a wrong way. Don't feel you can pick up the fine points on your own. Doing an exercise wrong is little better than not doing it at all; your muscles will not stretch and relax in the way they should, and your skill will not develop proportionately to the amount of time you put into it. Take classes, or ask an experienced friend to give you pointers. Form a group of friends and invite a teacher to one of your homes. When you take a class in any form of exercise, observe the teacher carefully *before* you imitate the movement. Remember to breathe. Holding the breath in a position of strain is damaging to your heart and prevents you from attaining flexibility. Think of your breath as the energy which propels your body.

Once you learn a calisthenic exercise well, you don't have to attend a class to do it but can squeeze it into whatever time spot is convenient for you.

Don't depend on others

Unless you play a sport which requires a partner, don't depend on friends to accompany you while you exercise. Though it may be enjoyable to have a friend jogging or swimming beside you, lending moral support and a friendly spirit of competition to the exercise, you musn't let your jogging or swimming session depend on the presence of that friend. If he or she stayed up too late the night before or has an unexpected engagement, go alone. You will find there is a meditative pleasure to exercising alone. As you jog, swim, or do yoga, you will be able to review your major concerns in your mind, concentrate totally on your exercise and the feeling it gives you, or daydream. A friend can sometimes distract you from the mood you want to indulge while you exercise.

Think positively

When you first begin to exercise, you will have to exert willpower to get yourself to do it. Your body and mind will heartily resist leaving your comfy armchair or mattress for the ardors of the swimming pool or exercise class. You can help yourself by not projecting negative images onto your workout session, such as, "The water will be so cold," "It's going to drizzle and I'll get wet and catch pneumonia," or "I'll feel exhausted afterward." Just get your body there. If every time you had to do any job, you thought in advance what a miserable experience awaited you, you would probably spend your life in bed.

Plan ahead

Your ultimate goal is to make exercise a ritual which will obtain a permanent place in your life. To do this, you have to plan ahead. Don't count on whims, invitations, or inspirations to get you to exercise. Schedule exercise into your daily activities with foresight. You may occasionally have to sacrifice. If you want to jog in the morning, for example, you will not be able to burn the candle until 4 A.M. If your afternoon dance class begins at five, regard that as a responsibility equivalent to getting to work in the morning or cooking dinner for the children. Don't let unexpected events interfere. Be firm. When you are invited to a dinner party on gymnastics night, arrive a bit late. Perhaps you will not be quite as well groomed when you rush to a social engagement after your swim or dance class, but you will be more relaxed and have a vital glow,

Body Exercises
103

more engaging than the three layers of fingernail polish you would have skipped your exercise session to apply.

Whenever you plan to exercise, it helps to have your equipment and what you will wear readily available. The biggest obstacle I know to a morning jogging session is having to grovel through the dirty laundry for a T-shirt and sweat pants or crawl under the bed to wrest your sneakers away from the dog.

Learn to use exercise as a psychic release

Exercising regularly provides you with an insurance policy against distress. When things go wrong in your life it helps to know that "What I need now is a good game of tennis" instead of "What I need now is a whiskey and soda." Exercise offers you an opportunity for psychic release which is not self-destructive. After my divorce, a good swim was the only activity which afforded me any relief, albeit temporary. I have one friend who jogs four miles, screaming, when she feels frustrated with her boss. If exercise is not already a well-established routine in your life, however, it cannot serve you when you feel angry or depressed. It is impossible to start moving your body for the first time when you are in the throes of despair. You need to know in advance that exercise will make you feel better.

Move more

Although no informal exercise can be substituted for a strenuous exercise, sport, or calisthenic, anytime you are able to move vigorously instead of remaining sedentary, you improve your health and vitality and augment the effects of your regular exercise session. Try bicycling to work instead of driving or taking public transportation. Climb stairs instead of using the elevator. When you walk, do so as vigorously as possible. Every morning I walk my dog, Carl, for half an hour in Central Park. But instead of merely plodding along, half asleep, I walk as rapidly as possible. I run a little, throw Carl's ball, and climb rocks. As I walk, I tighten the muscles of my buttocks and do my facial exercises. All this movement gets my blood flowing and prepares me for my day at work better than a sedentary hour spent over a cup of coffee and the newspaper.

BODY EXERCISES FOR YOUR FACE

As I stated earlier in this chapter, all physical exercise will improve the appearance of your face. I have designed several specific exercises, however, which are excellent for relaxing the face, filling it with color and animation, and improving, at the same time, the flexibility and strength of the back and neck. The condition of the spine, in fact, is closely related to the way the entire body looks and feels.

These five exercises should not become a substitute for your regular exercise routine; rather, they may be done in the morning, right after rising, just before you do your facial exercises or before a social or business engagement when it is important for you to look and feel alert and relaxed.

Forward and backward relaxes

Stand with your legs parallel about three feet apart. Bend over and relax forward. Make this movement easily, without strain. Touch the floor in front of you, bending your knees and back.

Then, relax backward, letting your arms drop in back of your thighs and hang down. Let your whole body relax and slump backward. Your head should hang and your knees should be bent. Don't straighten your knees as you change from the forward to the backward position. In both positions let the head and neck swing back and forth, and bounce your body and head. Swing down, bounce, bounce, then swing back, bounce, bounce. Repeat three to six times. These relaxes loosen the muscles in your head, neck, and waist, and as they do so they relax your face.

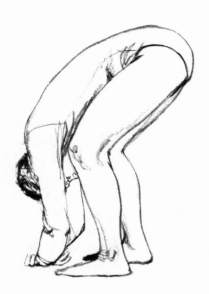

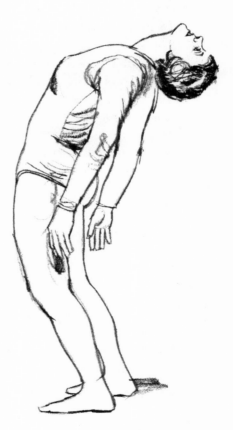

Body Exercises
107

Curving the neck, head, and spine

Sit on the floor with your legs crossed. Bend your head down toward your navel, keeping it as close to the center of your body as possible. The lower part of your spine should be straight. At first your head will only drop a short distance. Don't bounce or force your head downward. The feeling is not altogether pleasant in the beginning because your tight muscles don't want to let go. Concentrate on releasing the muscles in your neck and the upper part of your spine. Breathe deeply. As you exhale, feel your head drop farther toward your navel. This exercise relaxes the muscles in your neck and back, as shown by the side view, and releases the tension that has accumulated there. Your face will feel and look more serene and relaxed afterward. Spend two or three minutes on the exercise.

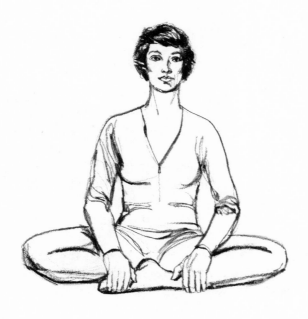

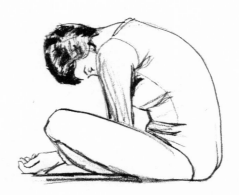

Aligning the head with the spine

Stand in front of a wall with your knees slightly bent. Bend over so that your head hangs toward your knees. Then straighten up slowly, pressing your back, vertebra by vertebra, into the wall. After you have done so, straighten your knees slowly. Use your stomach muscles to push the vertebrae of your lower back into the wall. Make sure all your vertebrae, from the lower part of the spine to the neck, are pressed against the wall. Repeat six times. This exercise improves your posture and firms your stomach muscles as it aligns the back with the neck and head. You should attempt to preserve this feeling of alignment when you walk and sit in your daily activities. As your posture improves, much of the tension in the back and neck, which is reflected in the face, is removed. Improved posture also flattens the stomach.

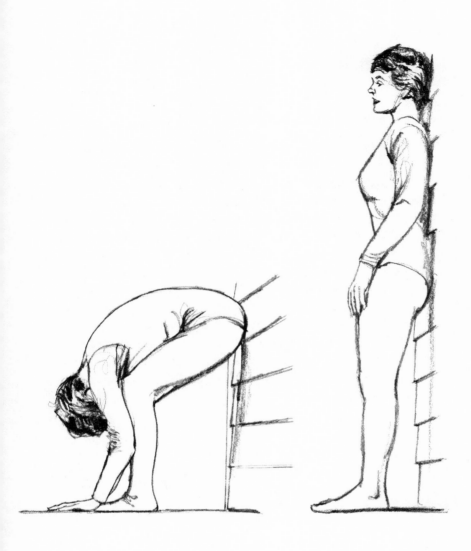

Bouncing the arms, shoulders, and back

Sit on the floor and lean against a low piece of furniture, like a bed or bench, which hits you about the middle of the shoulder blades. Pull your legs close to your body and rest your head on your knees. Slowly raise your head until it sits directly on top of your neck. Your entire back should be straight. Keep breathing. Now, raise your arms straight up, not back, and, keeping your back straight, lean back and bounce your arms and shoulders back. The work it takes to make this bouncing motion occurs mainly in your shoulders. Bounce ten times. Hang your body forward again and rest your head on your knees. This exercise is excellent for reducing tension in the upper back and shoulders. Practice releasing the muscles in your shoulders, head, and neck while your back is straight.

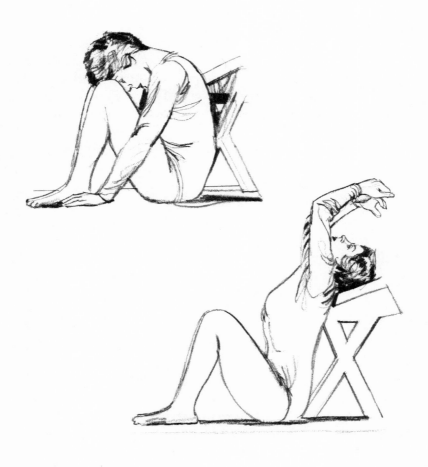

Headstand

If you can do a complete headstand, you are doing the best possible exercise for stretching the neck and spine and bringing blood to the face and head. Yoga experts tell us that the headstand brings blood to the brain, as well.

Many people feel that standing on the head is frightening, perhaps impossible. In my opinion, it is not nearly as hard as it looks. You must learn it from a qualified teacher, however, because if you do it incorrectly you are apt to injure yourself. Following are two alternative exercises which give you many of the same benefits as the full headstand. They are easy to do and involve no danger.

TRIANGLE HEADSTAND. Sit on your knees and put your hands on the floor, about a foot apart, with your fingers spread wide. The tips of your fingers should dig into the floor. Now, put your head down on the floor in front of your hands so that your hands and head form a triangle. The tip of your head should rest on the floor. Raise your knees and allow only your toes to rest on the floor. Walk in with your legs and get your feet as close to your hands as possible. This is the first stage of the headstand; it will stretch your neck and bring color to your face. Remain in the position as long as you can comfortably.

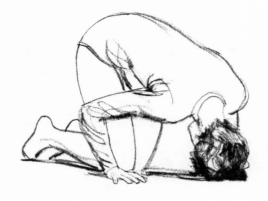

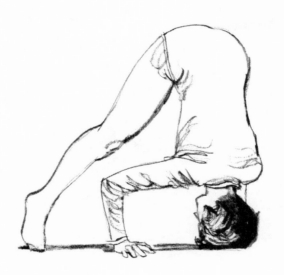

ALTERNATIVE HEADSTAND. Sit on your heels. Intertwine your fingers behind your back and lower your head to your knees. Rest your eyes on your knees. Raise your arms and hands, still intertwined, vertically above your back as your head touches your knees. Remain in the position as long as you can. This exercise stretches your arms and back and brings blood to the face. Raise your arms as high as possible and press your palms together. This is harder than it looks in the illustrations.

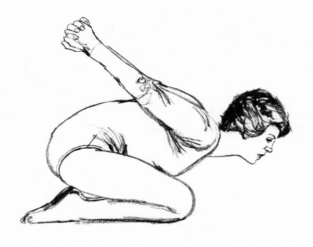

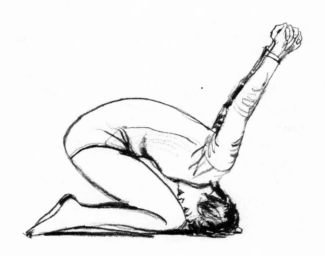

5 *The Facelift Diet*

Unfortunately, there is no magical combination of foods that will remove wrinkles and restore the bloom of youth to an aging face, any more than there is a fountain of youth with instantly rejuvenating waters. The diet that keeps your face taut, its skin elastic, and its outlines distinct is the same low-calorie diet that ensures you a slender, healthy, and vigorous body. A "facelift diet," then, is not really a diet at all, but a balanced regimen of nutritious foods which excludes those three *bêtes noires* guaranteed, in quantity, to pile on pounds—sugar, starches, and fats.

BINGE-DIET-BINGE CYCLES

The word diet for most of us describes a temporary period of deprivation—a month or two in which we bitterly replace large portions of our favorite foods with a Spartan intake of unsatisfying fare. Articles and books galore describe such diets, which promise to remove excess pounds rapidly through revolutionary means if only we can stick them out. Many advocate a limited number of foods in peculiar combinations: all the meat you want plus gallons of water, all the grapefruit you want, all the liver and hardboiled eggs and wine you want, or nothing but liquid protein. No longer in style is the old-fashioned reducing diet which permitted the overweight to eat small portions of many foods and shed pounds slowly, without depleting the body's nutrients.

The new "crash" diets, designed to tear the fat from the body, are nauseating, unsatisfying, trying to our nerves, and sometimes dangerous to health. The reason most of us put ourselves through them is that we know they will not last long. What we secretly think as we embark on our third day of Dr. Stillman's torture treatment is, "Soon I'll knock off that ten pounds and then I can eat normally again." And eat we do. At first we are cautious, but then we make excuses and cram our bottomless pits full of the delicious Danishes, fettucine, pecan pies, thick steaks, and potatoes au gratin we crave. Soon we take a disgusted look at our wobbling thighs and bulging stomachs and strain to zipper our pants and skirts, and we are searching for another revolutionary diet to rid ourselves of ten or twenty pounds again. Binge-Diet-Binge—it's a vicious circle.

What we fail to consider is that when we eat "normally" we eat too much. Our conception of a normal caloric intake is based on the amount and type of food we could consume at age eighteen without getting fat. For better or worse, as we near the middle of our lives—our bodies tell us when—we must decrease the amount of calories we consume by at least a third to maintain youthful figures and faces. This decrease in calories must be permanent. As you near forty the crash diet is out, and what I call a "sustaining diet" must take its place.

A sustaining diet is a comfortable plan to stabilize your body weight, an individualized regimen you must discover yourself and tailor to suit your needs. Whatever you decide to eat on a sustaining diet, however, you must prepare to sacrifice the majority of fattening foods you think you love—for life. This difficult prospect may become easier as you learn what the binge-diet-binge cycle does to your face.

HOW A CRASH DIET RUINS YOUR FACE

Although a few weeks on steak and water may have relatively little effect on your body and face when you are young, as you grow older the results can be disastrous. To understand why, visualize the flesh that lies beneath the skin of your face and neck as a piece of meat marbled with lines of fat. When you crash-diet, the fat is rapidly drawn away from deposits in various parts of the body and is processed in the bloodstream. Unfortunately, fat does not always cooperate by vanishing first from the places where your surplus is most apparent. You may lose fat quickly from your face and neck, while your over-padded hips remain intact.

The drastic reducing diet draws out the thin lines of fat from the face, creating empty channels and pockets, or wrinkles and sags. If you continue to starve yourself, the body may draw fat from the flesh itself, which causes the face to lose its structure. If you notice this unfortunate result and begin to eat "normally" again (i.e., too much), those empty channels are not necessarily refilled with fat. The fat you have dieted out of your face is difficult to replace in the same spot, and you will simply end up with more fat where you don't need it. Though your face may regain fat too, the wrinkles caused by each diet will remain. After years of a diet-binge-diet cycle, the skin of your face will become as stretched and empty as a deflated balloon.

The starvation diet contributes to an aged appearance in other ways. Because you feel deprived while dieting, you become cranky, with a tense, irritable expression—scarcely appealing or young. This mood change is produced partly because the fat which cushions your nerves against shock is also depleted. Well-meaning friends who advise you to stop dieting because you look "painfully thin" are not focusing on your large hips and wobbling thighs but on your drawn and haggard face.

Moreover, as your limited diet deprives your body of food elements necessary for its nutrition, the body will raid its own cells to get the vitamins, minerals, and proteins it needs to function. One of the reasons we age is that body cells fail to reproduce themselves. This will occur no matter what you eat, but if you deprive your body cells of the chemicals they need to reproduce for any period of time, you will speed up the aging process. The one way, then, to keep diets from playing havoc with your body and face is to maintain your body weight. Stop starving and then bingeing again.

WHY BE THIN?

Even in an age when most people admire a streamlined look, there is still a Victorian charm to the plump young face, smooth skinned and rosy. As that same plump face ages, however, its layers of fat cause it to lose its charm. When the skin of the face becomes noticeably lined, excess fat makes it look older. The fat on an older face tends to form pouches and bags which merge the face with the neck and give a puffy, bloated look. Fat blurs a face's distinctive outlines—its expressions, lines, and features—beneath unattractive padding. A fat old face, then, loses its individuality, the unique qualities a full life has put there.

I feel that if you are overweight, no matter what your age, it is better to diet, despite the risk of sags and wrinkles. If you lose the extra pounds through a sensible reducing diet (I favor a Weight Watchers-type program) over a long period of time and accompany your diet with exercise, your body tissue will not lose elasticity to the degree it would on a starvation diet. Even if some sags and wrinkles result, regular practice of my facial exercises will help your face regain its contours. In fact, as I mentioned earlier, I developed these exercises to replace the muscle tone I had lost in my own face after a crash diet. Your new, thin face will not only look younger but will portray your inner life more accurately. A thin body, needless to say, looks younger too. Without a protruding stomach and inhibiting fat, you fit into youthful clothing styles and move with greater agility.

The easiest way out of the binge-diet-binge cycle, of course, is to renounce vanity. "I'm past the age where looks are important," you might say. "I'd rather enjoy life, eat what I want, and be fat, jolly, and comfortable." This, in my opinion, is a serious cop-out. First, I doubt that overweight people really enjoy *life*. They may enjoy eating, but there's more to life than that. Their excess baggage prevents them from moving, dancing, and engaging in sports with ease and grace. The overweight tend to become sedentary, slow, and lazy; they observe more and participate less. Second, if the desire to look more attractive does not compel you to lose weight, health considerations should.

The same overly rich, refined diet that puts on pounds causes cholesterol level and blood pressure to rise. The heart must work harder to pump blood when you are fat, and as a result blood circulation is impaired. Cardiovascular diseases may result, as well as other chronic ailments. Many doctors and nutritionists believe that a number of health problems are caused by excess fats, refined flour, and sugar in the diet. Gerontologists say that reduced food intake may increase your chances of living longer. In short, if you don't love yourself enough to be vain, you owe it to those who do love you to be thin.

WHY WE OVEREAT

Most of us would like to be thin and yet 90 percent of Americans are fat. It is no news to most of us that the thinner we are, the more attractive and healthy we are; yet we contemplate our five, ten, fifteen, or more extra pounds with loathing, watch our stomachs bulging over our waistbands, our hips spreading beyond the boundaries of our slacks, and continue to overeat.

Nothing I have said so far about diet is news to anyone. We all know that lean meat, fresh vegetables, and salads are not fattening, and ice cream, cookies, and spaghetti are. We read about new diets all the time. We buy calorie counters and learn that a handful of nuts has 300 and three donuts have 525. We know that when we down a rich meal we will gain pounds, and that knowledge makes us feel guilty before, during, and after we eat it. We know that if we eat fattening foods at all, we should eat them in moderation. Yet, when presented with the opportunity to consume a sugar-, starch-, or fat-loaded tidbit, we wolf it down to the last morsel, and if no one presents us with such a treat, we manage to find it for ourselves. We exchange diets with each other, read books on dieting, collect menus that feature nonfattening foods, and yet return time and again to the box of cookies, the cheesecake for dessert, and the slice of bread between meals.

How many of us have sworn, "I'll eat this donut now and then I won't have dinner." And then, because someone invites us, we eat dinner too, complete with cheese hors d'oeuvres, a cocktail, and a slice of pie for dessert. Although we live in the most diet-conscious country in the world, we all continue to eat and stuff and despise ourselves for it, starve, then eat again. We all know that with even a moderate sense of discipline we can easily banish ten pounds and keep them away. We all know how to go about losing weight, and yet we continue to lose it, gain it back, and cry about the way we look. Why?

In part, we can blame our binge-diet-binge pattern on our society's schizophrenic attitude toward food—an attitude most of us reflect in our eating habits. On one hand, we uphold the skinny, athletic body as an aesthetic ideal. When we open a fashion magazine, we are confronted with only gaunt, hollow-cheeked models, for whom, it seems, all stylish clothing is designed. TV commercials and programs never feature rotund actors or actresses unless their very appearance is supposed to make us laugh. The personalities we are encouraged to admire for their elegance are always slender. Thus we are constantly informed by the media that to be beautiful is to be thin.

On the other hand, the same media sources that imbue us with this aesthetic ideal perpetuate our desire for fattening foods. The slender, athletic actors and actresses we see in TV commercials are more often than not advising us of the delights of a delicious, chocolately, coconut Mounds or the satisfying pleasure of a Budweiser beer. Magazines show us the latest fashions on skinny bodies and present us with a new crash diet every month, cheek by jowl with recipes for mouth-watering entrées and restaurant reviews.

Food as a temptation

Not only the idea of food but food itself constantly tempts us to eat. Throughout the country specialty food stores abound. Department stores display edible delicacies in a special section, so we can't even shop for a dress or a chair without thinking about our stomachs. There are restaurants everywhere, serving enormous portions— the one-pound steak or all-you-can-eat. Pizza chains, fried-chicken chains, hamburger houses galore, Dial-A-Steak, Blimpie Bases, and Dunkin' Donuts besiege us wherever we walk or drive. Our digestive juices, then, are constantly set aflow. In this land of plenty, whatever we want is readily available, and most of us can afford to feed ourselves with any food we crave.

Even when we try to resist temptation, food will not leave us alone. It follows us everywhere, forcing us to renounce our resolve. The hostess at a dinner party inevitably presents us with antidiet fare. We feel we will offend her if we refuse to partake heartily of the food she has labored to prepare. Besides, any excuse to abandon our distasteful diet is a good one and in we plunge. We say we eat to please her, but we eat when she is not looking too. In a restaurant it takes more character than we have to pay for a full meal and then decline the soup, warm bread, and dessert that comes with it. If we take a cruise where passage entitles us to six meals a day—including a midnight snack after a seven-course dinner—we eat all six meals because we paid for them.

Food as a celebration

To make matters worse, eating is one of the most important ceremonies of our lives. In this respect America is not unique. Joys, friendships, and sorrows are everywhere celebrated with food. When we meet friends it is always for a cocktail, lunch, dinner, or a cup of coffee (with a sweet)—we seldom meet just to chat without stuffing something into our mouths. All our rites of passage—weddings, Bar Mitzvahs, even funerals—are accompanied by food, not just a modest meal but an elaborate spread of gorgeous delicacies. We judge the host and the occasion by the amount and quality of food provided.

Food is always available, then, and we automatically eat whether we are hungry or not. After generations in the land of plenty, we still eat with the starved consciousness of our immigrant forebears, who came to the New World to escape a continent where food had become scarce. And while we are stuffing ourselves as if we had just stepped off the *Mayflower,* we have firmly in mind an image of how we would like to look—not the image our eating habits suggest (a plump Victorian with two chins) but the gaunt model in a *Vogue* magazine. Paradoxically, in countries where people actually starve, like India, to be beautiful is to be fat.

We perpetuate our cultural eating patterns by teaching our children what our parents taught us. The stereotype Jewish mother, who encourages her offspring to "have a little something" even when they are not hungry, is hardly confined to the Jews. As children we are all reminded of the starving children in Asia when we fail to clean our plates and are scolded for wasting food. When children cry, their parents offer them sweets, which they soon learn are supposed to cheer them up. We reward children for eating lima beans with extra dessert, but who was ever given an extra lima bean for finishing ice cream? The climax of a children's birthday party is a pink, sugary cake. When children visit a bank or gas station with their parents, the well-meaning institution presents them with lollipops. In short, from an early age we get the message that eating as much as possible is good for us and that the best, most rewarding food is sweet.

When we become adults we find sophisticated excuses to continue to indulge this childhood pattern. Modern psychology has given us a profound theory to employ as a rationale for stuffing ourselves called "oral gratification." The oral-gratification theory tells us that when we overeat it's because we are depressed, angry, starved for love, or confused. Thus a heavy day at the office, a memory of our mother's neglect, a phone call we didn't get, a spat with a loved one, bereavement, and boredom all make us forget our figures and appease our inner tumult with food. Needless to say, we would never dream of calming our rages and passions with a salad; nothing less than a banana split or an entire box of cookies will suffice. Logically, we know it is both inappropriate and ineffective to deal with our hearts through our stomachs— but we do.

There is a monolithic conspiracy, then, that keeps us

from having the slim shapes we desire. Our society's constant emphasis on food, plus the bad dietary patterns we learn in childhood, makes it a heroic task, both physically and psychically demanding, to stick to diets that keep us feeling healthy and looking young.

HOW TO STAY THIN

Resisting our favorite foods when a food-oriented society dangles them constantly before us calls for a revolutionary change in our eating attitudes. We must develop new concepts and new awarenesses about food and at the same time devalue its role in our emotional lives—a contradictory mission.

In order to develop a permanent sustaining diet, you must tailor a system of nourishing your body to your own metabolism, life-style, and taste buds. You must embark on a long process of discovery, look inward and outward, discard some of your lifelong notions about what to eat and when, what tastes good and what doesn't, and acquire new eating habits which you find pleasurable. Forget about finding the perfect diet in a magazine to dictate exactly what you should eat—that is someone else's system, not yours. Give yourself credit for being a unique individual, with your own psyche and body chemistry. The diet that keeps pounds off someone else's waistline is not guaranteed to keep pounds off yours. Following are my general suggestions on how to develop a sustaining diet and stay thin; some of them will apply to you and others will not. They are meant to be open-ended, to demonstrate the deep thought and planning necessary to permanently change your attitudes toward food, because, in case you have any doubts, staying thin is *work.* There's no way around it. Getting rid of a potbelly, bulging hips, and a fat face that took years to acquire cannot be done easily or overnight.

Make a decision

If you need to lose a great many pounds, your diet will have to be Spartan until they are gone—but it should include a variety of nourishing foods in small portions. Weight loss should be slow. Once the excess pounds are off, however, you are still faced with the prospect of eliminating fattening food from your diet on a permanent basis. If you truly love sugar, starches, and fats, there is no point minimizing the difficulty you will have renouncing them—especially for more than a short time.

Willpower and sacrifice are required. You must decide to pass up the goodies you adore with the same sense of dutiful resignation with which you would quit an interesting job that didn't pay a living wage or give up a lover who, despite his attractive qualities, made you miserable. You must truly want to be thin and healthy and must stay in touch with this ultimate goal. The decision to be thin cannot be halfhearted, temporary, or insincere. You must regard your decision as binding.

The interesting factor about binding decisions is that once they are made, whatever you have decided becomes easier to accomplish. There is no longer an inner conflict. You needn't ask yourself, "Should I have that cookie or not?" because you have already given the answer in advance. You will be called upon time and again, however, to exercise your willpower and reapply your decision to the temptation at hand.

Several years ago, for example, I took a cruise on the luxurious *France.* Because I was several pounds overweight and well knew what disastrous effects a seven-meal-a-day cruise could have on my waistline, I decided in advance not to touch a croissant, any bread, or rich desserts. Every morning when I went to breakfast the rich, buttery, warm croissants served with gooseberry jam were waiting to test my resolve. You can image how difficult it was to pass them up, but I did. I had decided that eating only one would invalidate my entire decision to diet.

Every morning I entered that dining room suffering the tortures of the damned. Would I be able to keep from having a single one of those heavenly croissants? And then I gritted my teeth, remembered my decision, and held out. I ordered a grapefruit, a soft-boiled egg, a Finn Crisp, and coffee while the concerned waiter stared at me with sad Gallic eyes. Once I had sat down and begun to chat with my tablemates, however, the croissant conflict vanished. I had successfully decided not to eat them, and believe me, I never gave them another thought—until the following morning. I lost weight on that cruise, and exercising my willpower gave me a feeling of self-admiration and strength. I did not regret giving up those croissants. In fact, I have regretted eating fattening foods, but I have never regretted resisting them.

Get in touch with hunger

The Zen Buddhists maintain that the greatest happiness is to eat when you're hungry and drink when you're thirsty. How many of us, however, can actually distinguish real hunger from a ravenous lust for food? When our eyes see something appetizing, it seems we feel instantly hungry. We think, "It's been four hours since I've had anything to eat," and we automatically assume that we are starved. When you feel the need for a between-meal snack, ask yourself if you're really hungry or if you only *think* you're hungry. Consider physiological factors: You may feel starved before dinner because you have relaxed after a hectic day or because you've skipped lunch, not because you have been doing the strenuous labor that makes one really hungry.

When you first switch from a diet of pastas, fattening cream sauces, and rich desserts to a piece of broiled fish, fresh asparagus spears, and a pear, your whole body will protest. You may feel light-headed, faint, nauseated, or sleepy. Don't worry, you are not starving, but your emotions are fooling you with false signs of hunger. Concentrate on the nausea, the headache, the sleepy feeling. Tell yourself why these conditions are occurring, and they will vanish soon. I always feel happy when I'm really hungry because I know then that I'm losing weight.

Learn to question your appetite for particular foods as well. When you succumb to temptation and cut a slice of cheesecake or some other high-calorie treat, ask yourself before you shovel it in, "Do I really want this cheesecake?" After every bite, ask yourself, "Am I really enjoying this cake?" Chew it slowly and thoughtfully. Is it really *that* wonderful, or do you just assume it is because you have always thought so? I have found, to my surprise, that after a period of abstention from fattening foods, those starchy, sugary goodies I thought I craved did not taste quite as delicious as I had remembered but rather dry and artificial. My taste buds had readjusted to the natural sugar and fresh, clean taste of the melon and fruit I'd been eating for dessert instead. Whether a certain food tastes fantastic or not is largely an acculturated idea. Present a primitive man in a Brazilian jungle with a piece of cheesecake and he would undoubtedly spit it out.

Learn new ways to prepare low-calorie foods

When most people consider eliminating fattening foods from their diets, they contemplate a barren wasteland of meals they find boring, tasteless, and unsatisfying. We can make an endless list of foods we cannot eat and remain thin, because sugar, starch, and fat, alone and in combination, encompass all the goodies we think we love. In short, we feel condemned either to a hell of broiled fish, boiled vegetables, and a little fruit or to a heaven of cakes, pies, pastas, and roast beef Wellington, which we pay for with fat. Considering this outlook, it's not surprising that we should be secretly planning our next binge as we knock off a few pounds with a distasteful diet.

In order to enjoy nonfattening food you must learn to make it appetizing from your point of view. There is more than one way to prepare a low-calorie meal. Lean meat with a vegetable does not necessarily signify bland, tasteless fare. Discover new ways to use spices, seasonings, and marinades. A broiled chicken, for instance, can be vastly improved by rubbing powdered ginger, salt, pepper, and lemon juice into the skin before cooking. Fish can be intriguing when baked in wine. Study vegetarian cookbooks and discover new ways to cook natural foods. Experiment with Indian, Japanese, and Chinese cuisines.

With some imagination you can also discover nonfattening ways to prepare your favorite fattening recipes. For example, you may substitute low-calorie yogurt for sour cream in most recipes without an appreciable difference in taste. On the other hand, a touch of a mildly fattening sauce can satisfy your craving for a rich meal. I often make a green sauce, which consists of mayonnaise, a little watercress, and a few tablespoons of milk blended with whatever fresh herbs my greengrocer has available. A tablespoon of this tangy sauce (100 calories) transforms an otherwise dreary portion of broiled fish or chicken into a gourmet delight.

This process of experiment and discovery should redirect some of the energy you invest in eating into constructive channels and challenge your creativity as well. Instead of devoting so much time to the spiritual question, "Should I have that strawberry shortcake or not?", find interesting ways to avoid that question altogether.

Make a ceremony of eating less

Even small portions of low-calorie foods can be served magnificently and eaten with style. Focus more energy on the way you eat. Don't grab or eat standing up or on the run; sit down, relax, and concentrate on the atmosphere of the meal. Chew your food slowly and relish it instead of assuming that because it's not fattening, it's not delicious either. When you eat quickly, the amount and type of food you consume gets lost in the gobbling process.

Bring all your five senses to a meal to make it most enjoyable. Set the table with your finest linen, china, and silver. Dine by candlelight, even when dining alone. Eat one night a week in a Japanese restaurant, where small portions of low-calorie foods are served with traditional artistic elegance. When you broil a fish, take the time to garnish it with parsley or dill. Prepare a gorgeous salad or fruit cup, making the most of the vivid colors nature offers. Smell the aromas, enjoy the colors and textures of the food as well as the taste.

Fast

When you eat, make the most of it; at other times you may want to stop eating altogether. Some people maintain their weight by observing periods of total abstinence. One friend of mine fasts on water one day a week. Another spends two days on an all-liquid diet. She recommends buying an electric juicer; there is no low-calorie food, she swears, as delicious and satisfying as a glass of fresh carrot juice. Partial fasts are also possible. I often finesse meat and carbohydrates and eat three large all-vegetable meals several days a week.

Skipping meals is another form of fasting. Although American nutritionists tell us breakfast is the most important meal of the day, I feel it's a mistake to eat in the morning, or anytime, if you're not hungry. If you don't feel like breakfast, don't eat until lunch; that first meal may merely open up the stomach for business. If you skip a meal, however, don't make up for it by tripling your usual intake at the next one.

Although it is generally inadvisable to substitute snacks for meals when weight watching, some people find this the best method for reducing overall calorie consumption. Make sure snacks are filling and nutritious.

Plan ahead

In order to stick to a sustaining diet, you must conscientiously study your body's needs for food and prepare to meet them. Ask yourself when you feel most hungry and know in advance what you will eat at that time. Don't abandon your appetite to fate. Resistance to the food you should not eat breaks down easily when you're starved and there's no low-calorie food available. If hunger pangs attack you regularly at 11 A.M., and you are inclined to run like a ravenous wolf for the coffee wagon's cheese Danish tray, bring an apple to work. If you know you'll be starved after a morning of shopping, tote a plastic container of tuna salad to eat in a park. Check out restaurants near your office or favorite haunts and discover which ones serve good soups, salads, and other low-calorie fare. When you're on the run, fattening snacks are the easiest ones to grab; be prepared.

We often get ready for a dinner party where the hostess is likely to serve a gargantuan feast by fasting all that day. By evening we're starved and upset the balance of our diet by consuming an abnormally large meal. The following morning, instead of feeling sated, we are ravenous again. Although experts say it is physically impossible to "stretch" the stomach with too much food, most of us have experienced this phenomenon. Perhaps what we stretch is our desire for food. In any case, I would advise facing a dinner party not by "emptying out" but by eating as you usually do all day and having a hard-boiled egg just before the feast. Eggs expand and fill the stomach, making it difficult to eat as much rich food at the party.

Try visualizing as accurately as possible the meal you are apt to confront. Plan in advance exactly what you will eat and what you won't. Vow to yourself: I will have one hors d'oeuvre and one cocktail, two servings of meat and vegetable, no bread or potatoes, and perhaps one bite of dessert. Seeing the meal in your mind beforehand may lessen its visual appeal when you get there. You may find your imagination made the spread more tempting than it actually is.

Deal with emotions in new ways

Any plan for a sustaining diet faces its Waterloo during a bout of depression, grief, anxiety, or boredom. When a strong emotion supersedes your desire to be thin, it is hard to remember a sensible diet; you want to feel better as rapidly as possible. For many people feeling better is synonymous with eating. Our excuse as we head for the ice cream parlor is, "I can't help having this chocolate milk shake; I'm depressed. I deserve this milk shake." The implication is, "My depression caused me to eat this ice cream today, but tomorrow I will go back to eating normally." The problem with this theory, of course, is that tomorrow we may be depressed for another reason. Our emotional ups and downs will always be with us, and if we indulge them with food, so will our excess pounds. After an "oral-gratification" binge, most of us feel worse; the tempting morsel is gone and we can feel the pounds creeping on again, making us feel fat, ugly, and old— a cause for greater depression.

If you are inclined toward oral gratification, sit down and analyze the moods that compel you to eat. Plan, in advance, new ways to gratify yourself when these moods occur. Make a list of events that interest you, clothes you would like to own, whims you want to indulge, a beauty salon you have been wanting to visit. The next time you are depressed, anxious, or bored, or need to reward yourself, select an alternative gratification. I often buy flowers instead of food when I am depressed. Advance planning is important; when you're actually in the throes of a negative mood, it won't be as easy to dream up new ways to thwart an old, destructive habit.

Many people overeat when they are bored; some eat at a particular hour simply because they have always eaten at that time of day. To avoid these pitfalls, try filling the gaps you automatically fill with food with other activities. Study belly dancing, jog, swim, or take an exercise class during lunch hour. When you are home alone, bored, and inclined to reach for the potato chips, reach for the telephone, a pen, or knitting needles instead. When you are lonely, invite a friend to join you at the theater or the movies instead of at dinner. Plan ways to minimize the role of food in your life.

When you are about to succumb to oral gratification and pop a handful of cashews into your mouth, ask yourself, "Why am I eating these cashews?" If the honest answer is, "I'm eating them because I'm bored," you may feel silly enough to put the nuts back in the jar. Logically, we all know that eating will not make us feel happy, stimulated, or less lonely, but we tend to eat anyway during difficult periods, without being in touch with the reason why. Consider that eating may be a way to avoid the expression of emotion. When you eat you stuff the emotions down with the food instead of letting them out. If you're depressed, cry.

Employ visual aids

I am a great believer in visual aids. Place signs on the pantry door which say, "Stay thin!" or which note the number of calories in your favorite fattening foods. When my son diets he hangs a drawing of an obese man with the caption "Eat, Piggy" on the refrigerator door. Make a poster featuring a photo of yourself as you are side by side with a photo of a slimmer you. When you see someone eating a tempting dessert in a restaurant or a double-decker ice cream cone on the street, focus on the eater instead of his food; usually he will be overweight.

Nothing encourages me to stop eating more than the sight of an overweight man or woman eating too much.

Trick your body

Many people sustain body weight by making a firm decision to eliminate certain foods and sticking to it. Others with less powerful wills may need to devise ways to trick the body into renouncing its favorites until it becomes adjusted to new eating habits. There are endless tricks you can play.

If you are mad about sweets, for example, it may be false idealism to think you can renounce them forever. Try eating just one bite of dessert—this bite may satisfy your body's need for sugar without overloading it with 400 calories. But know thyself—one bite of confection may induce you to consume the entire cake. If you have always drunk coffee with cream and three teaspoons of sugar (about 100 calories), black coffee (0 calories) may be more bitter than your taste buds can bear. Lower the amount of sugar you use week by week, accustoming yourself to the new taste. When you finally stop using sugar completely, the black coffee will taste almost sweet.

As you wean yourself from pie and cake, eat an entire cantaloupe in their place, if necessary. A whole melon is still not as fattening as a piece of pie, and eventually you will be satisfied with less. If you yearn for starches, substitute imported flatbreads, like Finn Crisp, for raised bread. Three or four Finn Crisps have the same number of calories as one slice of bread; if you imagine each crisp *is* a slice of bread, you will feel more satisfied. If you aren't filled by small portions at first, drink a glass of water before the meal. Remember, your goal is to change your eating habits for life; allow for a period of adjustment.

STOP FOOLING YOURSELF

While you are fooling your body with new preparations of slimming foods and new eating habits, you must avoid fooling yourself. Even with the best intentions and the greatest determination, most of us find one excuse after another to break our diets and eat fattening foods. We don't consciously decide to start bingeing again but kid ourselves into believing that even while we are stuffing fattening morsels into our mouths, we are still sacrificing.

We constantly allow our minds to fool us with rationalizations. We pass a candy store and say, "I'll just have a few macadamia nuts. After all, they may be a bit fattening but they contain protein," or, "Tonight I won't have much dinner, just an apple, so now I can have a plate of spaghetti with butter sauce." We grab a hot dog with a roll for lunch because we didn't have time to sit down and order a salad; then we have an ice cream cone because everyone knows a hot dog isn't enough of a lunch. We sample one tiny cheese Danish from the new bakery and hope that it floats through our body unnoticed. We have a low-calorie dinner of broiled fish and vegetables but drink two martinis before, which we don't count because technically they're not food. Then we get on the scale and wonder how on earth we gained three pounds when we have deprived ourselves so severely. "I can't eat a thing without gaining weight," we say with a moan. "I must have a metabolic problem." Secretly we hope the doctor can prescribe a pill that will spirit our pounds away, so we can go on eating what we want.

Moreover, after we have gained weight, we delude ourselves into thinking that we're still thin. "I seem to be retaining water," we think as the pounds pile on, or we look at ourselves in a mirror and dismiss the bulges we see as a temporary mirage created by the garments we are wearing. The scale must be wrong, we think, and hop on another, which we judge to be wrong too. Although it is unrealistic to hope to attain the angular, breastless, hipless form of a nineteen-year-old *Vogue* model, you should not dismiss the five extra pounds on your derrière as an optical illusion. I have noticed that my friends over-react to every blemish they imagine ruins their faces, while they tend to overlook the ten pounds that really do damage their silhouettes. The reason is obvious: As long as they think they're thin, they can continue to overeat. How can you stop fooling yourself about what you eat? My first suggestion is to stand in front of a full-length mirror and take a good look; don't hide from yourself. Here are some others.

Monitor your food intake

If you want to stay thin, you must count and evaluate every morsel of food you put into your mouth. If you stick to your diet all day and then slip four cookies down the hatch before bedtime, you should not be surprised to find you haven't lost weight. The sad truth is that some people can eat cookies now and then and stay slim, and others can't.

If you don't own a scale, buy one and weigh yourself every morning. This practice will soon teach you how much food your body will absorb before expanding. Face the consequences of your eating habits immediately. If you seem to gain weight despite your diet, buy a calorie counter and tally the caloric value of all the food you eat every day. Buy a food scale and weigh portions, if necessary. You may find you've been deceiving yourself about the actual number of calories contained in different foods. Fruit, for example, is believed to be low in calories. Many fruits, however, contain 100 calories or more per 3½ ounces (bananas, apples, grapes, nectarines, and others) and should not be eaten in quantity. Liquids, too, contain calories—a small glass of orange juice has between 55 and 70.

Don't confuse "healthy" with "nonfattening" either. Seeds, nuts, brown rice, granolas, and dried fruits are loaded with calories. If you're going to have eight dates (200 calories), you might as well have the brownie (150 calories) you crave. Honey is actually more caloric than refined sugar.

If you know little about nutrition, buy a book and educate yourself. Find out which foods give you the most energy, vitamins, and protein with their calories.

Beware of "diet" foods

Although special dietary concoctions may not have many calories, they perpetuate the desire for the wrong kinds of food. My European friends find nothing more amusing than the American "diet" cookie—a cookie with nothing real or delicious in it, which is supposed to help you lose weight. When you're on a diet, you want to forget about cookies, not stimulate the memory of them with tasteless imitations. Diet sodas, too, keep you hankering after sweets. Try dismissing the idea of soda altogether, and drink Perrier mineral water with a dash of lemon instead. Many so-called diet foods are more fattening than you think. I'm sure you've heard, "Have a yogurt, it's not fattening." The truth is that while plain yogurt is low in calories, those with preserves in the bottom are as fattening as ice cream. Don't have something merely because it's not fattening; simply don't have it. Eat when you're hungry or not at all. Remember, too, that *anything* is fattening if you eat enough of it.

Don't buy food you shouldn't eat

The best way to avoid dredging a fattening snack out of the cupboard is not to have it there. Don't buy a bag of crumb buns, telling yourself you won't have a single one, or maybe just a bite. Who's kidding who? Don't buy cookies, candy, and ice cream "only for the children." You'll be tempted to eat them too. Children don't need fattening junk food any more than you do, and feeding it to them constantly and using it as a reward will only inflict your problem on them in later years. Try introducing milk shakes made with milk and fresh fruit and dried fruit and nuts to your children in place of artificial sweets. When you do buy ice cream for the children, buy enough for one serving only instead of several gallons that will beckon from the freezer for the next four weeks. Children may protest this change in policy for a while, but they will gradually grow accustomed to new treats.

Avoid unnecessary binges

All of us are human, and even the most determined dieter will lose control and eat a forbidden food now and then—a cookie, perhaps. If you've broken down and eaten a cookie, it's not the end of the world—and certainly no excuse to beat your breast with guilt and remorse and then finish off the entire box. Although you can't expect to change a lifetime of poor eating habits all at once, there's a difference between losing some control and taking advantage of a momentary lapse of discipline to run amuck.

The opportunity to binge will occur often, and sometimes binges are unavoidable, almost necessary, to preserve good social relations. Recently, for example, I was invited to the home of one of my college students. She had gone to great trouble and expense to prepare a five-course French meal which began with Quiche Lorraine and ended with carrot cake topped with whipped cream. I was the honored guest; it would have been insulting and bad manners for me not to eat what she served or even to rave about the weight I was gaining—so I forgot about my diet. Granted, I could have eaten smaller portions of her delicious food, but I didn't. I chalked it up to a "mandatory" binge.

There is a huge difference, however, between a binge sheer good manners force you to enjoy and the endless excuses you make and games you play with yourself in order to keep overeating. It may be in poor taste to resist the food a friend or loved one goes to great trouble to prepare, but you can resist bingeing at a buffet, where no one really notices what you eat anyway, or in a restaurant, where you can choose your meal. If you blow your diet now and then, it's not a catastrophe, but there is no reason to let a single orgiastic dinner party turn into a month of desserts, pastas, and hot rolls. If you succumb to a binge, return to your moderate diet immediately.

Although some excuses to binge are better than others, there's no excuse to sashay off the street into a candy store for a bag of chocolate marzipan creams because you feel depressed. After forty there's *nothing* in a candy store for you!

6 *Skin Care*

Until recently the primary focus of the cosmetics industry was on colorful powders, pastes, and pencils designed to heighten our good features and conceal our flaws. Now the emphasis has changed. We are a nation obsessed with skin care. Cosmetic companies all sport a line of expensive skin-treatment products—astringents, cleansing lotions, moisturizers, and masques. We have learned that the basis of an alluring face is not a cosmetic glaze but a clear, radiant skin beneath. A heavily painted face is out and the natural look is in—although, we are told, it takes a good many cosmetics to look properly "natural." Every magazine we read has at least one article on skin care. Books, famous personalities, and renowned dermatologists advise us how to clean and nourish the complexion, be it aging, oily, blemished, or dry.

This trend, I feel, is positive. In Europe chic women have always emphasized basic skin care more than a cosmetic coating. Most of New York's leading cosmetologists, in fact, are from eastern Europe, where many formulas for skin care were derived. The endless messages we receive on skin care, however, often contradict one another. Every dermatologist, it seems, has a different theory on what's good and what's bad for the skin, and every cosmetic company has another. When we read articles about skin care, we find no two of them give us exactly the same advice. In the end, if we tried every formula and theory these experts recommend, we would constantly be spending time and money on skin care concoctions and techniques, consuming large quantities of different vitamins, and, in the end, feeling more confused and looking about the same as we did before.

Most of us now know that it's important to clean skin properly, to moisturize it, and to protect it from damaging environmental influences. We all need a basic system to keep our complexions clean and fresh with a minimum expenditure of time and money. It is also important to realize that the best treatment we can give the skin does not come from an elegant jar. In my opinion, the ingredients that keep the skin alive and young are the same ingredients that keep our bodies fit and slender—good, nourishing food, rest, and exercise. The reason for this lies in the basic construction of the skin itself.

THE STRUCTURE OF THE SKIN*

The skin is more than an attractive wrapper; it is an organ of the body designed to protect the inner organs

*I am indebted to Dr. Bedford Shelmire, Jr.'s, *The Art of Looking Younger* (New York: St. Martin's Press, 1973) for my description of the physiology and aging of the skin in the two sections that follow.

from the environment and to seal necessary fluids in and harmful substances out. This organ consists of an external layer, the one we see, and a layer beneath it that we don't see.

The outer layer is composed of a thick sheet of cells. These living cells die and are then pushed to the surface of the skin by the new cells forming beneath them to take their place. The dead cells fall away, taking with them dirt and bacteria. When we wash the skin, we help it shed this layer of dead cells and, in the process, keep the skin clean and clear. The outer layer of the skin, too, contains pigment, which darkens to protect the inner layer when we are exposed to the sun. Superficial damage to the outer layer is easily repaired by the skin itself, which rapidly reconstructs its sheet of cells.

The vital layer of the skin, however, is the invisible inner layer, which cannot be replaced or regenerated; damage to it results in scar tissue or structural change. This layer, composed of an elastic type of tissue called collagen, is responsible for nourishing the skin, oiling it, cleaning out its wastes, and determining its general resilience and tone. A large portion of this task falls to the small blood vessels in the skin, which bring in food and water and remove wastes through channels called ducts. The more vigorous our blood circulation, the more rapidly the blood vessels of the skin do their nourishing and waste-removing job. The longer that waste remains in the skin, the more likely it is to blemish it. When waste hangs in, the chemicals that help the cells divide do not work as efficiently: fewer cells divide, meaning we have fewer new cells. Sweat glands in the skin also remove wastes. The oil glands, the ends of which we see in the form of pores, soften and protect the skin with sebum, or oil (not too much, we hope, or too little).

This description of the skin is simplified, but the message should be clear: The basic condition of the skin is determined largely by the inner layer, which is nourished and cleaned via the circulatory system, as is any organ. We can improve the efficiency of this system of nourishment and waste removal with exercise, which increases circulation, and with proper diet; these factors play a more important role in skin care than anything we can do to the outside of the skin.

WHAT HAPPENS TO THE SKIN AS WE AGE?

As we age, the outer layer of skin automatically becomes thicker and drier. A different kind of cell, shed less easily, is produced by older skin. This cell buildup coarsens the texture of the skin and makes the pores appear larger. The older cells hold less moisture than younger skin cells, so the skin becomes rougher and is spangled with superficial lines. The pigment of the skin, too, grows darker. Also, the production of hormones, which spur the function of the oil glands, decreases, and the skin loses much of its natural moisturizing cream. Women are especially affected by this hormonal decline, which becomes pronounced around the time of menopause.

The inner layer of skin ages, too. The collagen fibers which give the skin tone and elasticity break down, weakening the supporting tissue. Along with loss of muscle cells, this collagen breakdown causes wrinkles and grooves.

Unfortunately wrinkles are inevitable, and no human skin is immune to the effects of aging. Good nutrition, care, and lack of abuse, however, can prevent aging before it is due and help us preserve a smooth and lively skin, whether wrinkles crease it or not.

HOW TO AVOID PREMATURE AGING

Most of the practices which help preserve the inner layer of skin and prevent premature aging come in the form of *don'ts*.

Don't sunbathe

"Not again," you may say with a groan when you read "Don't sunbathe." For several years dermatologists and skin experts have been loudly proclaiming the negative effects of this popular practice; yet few of us want to hear about them or believe they are true. Nothing makes those of us who live in cities or in northern climates feel better during or after a freezing winter than exposing our chilled skin and bones to the sun's warming rays. Our complexions lose the unhealthy color of a trout's belly, and the sun imbues us with the radiant glow of youth and good health. We all believe a suntan makes us look beautiful, vital, and younger, and we try to stay in the sun as long as possible to prolong this wondrous transformation. Unfortunately, the positive effects of a sunbath are a deceptive illusion.

When exposed to the sun the skin's blood vessels expand, puffing out the skin and coloring it a rosy hue, which, unless you overbroil, looks superficially attractive. Wrinkles and grooves are partially concealed by the increased volume of the rest of the skin, so the puffing process makes you look younger. But don't forget that these initial, glowing stages of the suntan you crave are really the results of the swelling of your poor, overheated skin.

If you remain in the sun, the skin gathers its pigment and builds cells in thicker layers to provide a screen for the inner layer of skin. This is your tan. If you leave the sun after a few sessions of moderate exposure, you are still ahead, but if you continue to indulge in prolonged sunbaths, day after day, year after year, the temporary changes the sun creates in the skin become permanent; dark yellow or white areas of pigmentation and dilated blood vessels result, as well as damage to the blood vessels and the elastic fibers of the inner layer of skin. Often rough, scaly patches of skin develop—especially in those with fair complexions—and these are the precursors of skin cancer. These changes are cumulative; that is to say, overexposure to the sun from ages twenty-four to thirty-two are not negated by five summers of no exposure. The skin remembers and records the sun's damage. The result is that when natural effects of aging begin to take hold, all the permanent effects of sunbathing may appear at once, and owing to your sun worshiping you may look older overnight.

You may now be perfectly willing to swap ten years of looking dreadful when you've passed middle age for a few months of looking glorious when you're forty. Consider, however, that the positive effects of a suntan are temporary, at best. We look most attractive when we first expose ourselves to the sun. A painful burn is never enhancing, and a deep tan has a way of turning perversely yellow, flaky, and leathery the minute fall comes and you are forced indoors. As your tan fades and your normal skin tone is restored, you may find your skin dry, rougher than it was before, and possibly coarse and splotched. You may discover small, brown, wartlike growths on your body—another disagreeable evidence of aging and sun damage combined.

On the other hand, if sunbathing does make you feel like you look terrific—an important factor in actually looking good—limit your sunbathing to a few days a year, or, as the experts suggest, protect your skin with a good sunscreen containing PABA. Try sunbathing swathed in a light but tightly woven cotton caftan and a straw hat, which permit you to soak in those restorative rays while preserving your skin intact. Remember, there is a huge difference between brief bouts of sun worshiping on a beach in a northern climate and exposing yourself to the fiery rays of an equatorial sun in Miami or the Caribbean a few weeks a year or all year long. Consider, too, that it may not be the sun that makes you feel so good but the tranquilizing effect of fresh or salty air. If you do some form of strenuous exercise regularly, you will have a healthy color all year without the sun, and it will be the color of authentic good health, not a superficial, transitory glow.

Stop smoking and drinking to excess

Smoking damages the organs responsible for circulation—the heart and lungs—and also impairs blood flow to the skin, depriving it of oxygen. Experts tell us that smoking promotes wrinkling and coarse skin texture, particularly around the eyes. Look at any woman you know who has passed thirty-five and smokes excessively; then look at those who don't. You will see a noticeable difference in the smoker's skin; it is probably somewhat coarse and sallow, clearly gasping for a little air, and she may have crow's-feet around her eyes. If you are a smoker, a mirror may help you more than an x-ray of your lungs to quit this destructive habit.

Alcohol is a toxic substance, and excess consumption has a bad effect on the skin at any age. Anyone who drinks too much will suffer from an unhealthy, tired-looking skin. As you get older, however, these effects are more pronounced. In some people alcohol may cause the blood vessels in the face to become inflamed and break, creating small red lines and a mottled skin.

Don't massage your skin roughly

If you practice facial massage, do it gently. Pushing and pulling the skin of the face with too much force can damage the buttressing structure. If you want to stimulate the skin, try slapping it lightly. Never, never touch the skin beneath the eyelids, which is as delicate as the finest parchment and easy to stretch. When you apply cream to this area, do so with light pats; don't rub it in.

Don't burn the candle at both ends

Irregular sleeping hours are a prime cause of a sallow skin and a fatigued face. As we get older we can no longer stay up half the night and wake up looking anything other than haggard and worn. Circles under the eyes, lines and hollows in the face, and poor skin texture are all magnified by lack of sleep. Try to get to bed at approximately the same time every night and rise at a regular hour in the morning. Special occasions will occur that keep you up late, but don't make them a habit. If you suffer from insomnia, exercise, in my opinion, is the magical cure for all but the most stubborn cases.

The best way to nourish the skin is from the inside. As I said in chapter 5, nothing harms the inner structure of the skin more than a crash diet based on only a few foods, which may fail to provide the cells with the nutrients they need to reproduce and leaves sags and bags after weight loss. The diet that benefits the skin is a nourishing protein- and fiber-rich diet. My favorite skin food is liver. Super rich in many vitamins and proteins, liver is a lean meat and nonfattening (unlike beef, which contains many of the same vitamins and minerals). Some think that the vitamin Bs in liver help free the skin of excess oil and pigmentation. If you hate liver, try ordering it in a restaurant, where it will be appetizingly prepared and part of a special occasion.

I also believe in eating plenty of leafy green and fibrous vegetables such as spinach and carrots, which contain vitamin A, essential for keeping the texture of the skin smooth and preventing dryness and premature aging. Vitamin C, contained in citrus fruits and also (in small quantities) in green, leafy vegetables, helps the skin stay elastic and resist infection. Fruits and vegetables, as well as bran, contain fibers which aid waste elimination. Nothing clouds the complexion more than a severe case of constipation. If you have this problem, try to regulate it naturally with a high-fiber diet and lots of water; avoid laxatives.

IMPROVING THE SKIN WITH EXERCISE

If there is one magic word in this book it's *exercise*. I think it's worth repeating that nothing makes your entire body more beautiful and youthful than regular exercise.

What affects the rest of your body affects your skin. Exercise improves circulation, expands the blood vessels, brings oxygen to the skin, and helps remove wastes from it faster. The more you exercise, the cleaner and more glowing your complexion will be.

However much care and protection we give the inner layer of skin, the outer layer is the one we touch and see, the one we think about and, naturally, try to improve. Though the importance of creams, soaps, and astringents is to my mind somewhat exaggerated by the media, proper skin care can make a huge difference in the way our complexions appear to the world. We all need an efficient system of cleansing and moisturizing the skin with products that enhance rather than damage its positive qualities. Following are the important steps for effective skin care.

Recognizing your skin type

Skin types are as variable as individual personalities and may change with age, stress, the season, and the environment. Skin products are designed for different types of skin, and it is important to use the right products to avoid excess oil or dryness.

If you have oily skin, it absorbs makeup quickly and emits a thin, greasy film sometimes shortly after cleansing and upon waking in the morning. Dry skin reveals itself by a taut feeling after washing and small white flakes in the dry areas. Many people have combination skin, which is dry in some areas and oily in others. Realistically evaluate your own skin—with your eyes, not your mind. Cosmetic companies try to convince us that almost all skin older than twenty is about to wrinkle and needs moisturizers and creams to protect it. Actually, oily skin, even acne, is a common phenomenon in women well over thirty, who may suffer from the pore-clogging effects of extra oils. On the other hand, skin which has always been oily may become distinctly drier as we age or in response to central heating. Normal skin, never oily or dry, is rare. If you are having trouble evaluating your skin type, enlist the aid of a cosmetician. Be alert to changes in your skin and respond with appropriate skin products.

Cleansing properly

If your skin is perpetually oily, flaky, or tight, the chances are you are not cleansing it correctly with the proper product. Oily skins need drying soaps and should be washed often, though not excessively. If your skin is dry, you need a gentle, nondetergent soap (I prefer Nivea soap or Neutrogena) or a cleansing lotion that you can wash off with water. Whatever you wash your skin with, make sure you *get it off*. Any residue of soap or cleansing lotion allowed to remain on the skin clogs the pores and irritates the skin tissue. Some cosmeticians advise rinsing with thirty splashes of water. This may be a bit extreme, but make sure all traces of the cleansing agent are gone. Don't buy cleansing lotions with directions that advise you to leave them on the face. You may not want to wash your face with soap for fear of drying it, but water is the primary moisturizing agent of the skin and can never harm it.

When washing, avoid water that is too hot or icy cold. Extreme temperatures may dry the skin or excite oil glands and traumatize the skin's tiny blood vessels. Luke-warm water is best.

Don't be rough with a towel or washcloth and don't scrub or rub. This won't aid cleaning or drying and may stretch skin tissue.

Deep cleansing and exfoliation

No matter what type of skin you have, it needs—oc-casionally or often—a deep cleansing, which helps the skin shed its layer of dull, dead cells and accumulations of debris in the pores. As you grow older and your skin's cells shed less easily of their own accord, this exfoliation process becomes more important.

If your skin is dry, close-pored, and delicate, you may only need to undertake this process once every two weeks. Large-pored, oily skins, prone to pimples and blackheads, may need a deep cleansing every few days. You may use one or all of the following methods to deep-clean your skin.

FACIAL SAUNA. Some dermatologists and cosme-ticians recommend a facial sauna, or a steam treatment, which opens the pores, causes the skin to sweat and rid it-self of wastes, and promotes circulation. Others feel a sauna is basically useless and may dry and irritate the skin.

There are commercial saunas, but you can make your own version by heating some water to the boiling point, removing the lid from the pot, then making a tent out of a towel or sheet to cover your head and the pot. The tent traps the steam. If the steam feels too hot, let the pot cool for a while. Be sure to wear sunglasses or goggles to protect the delicate skin around your eyes. I add two tablespoons of camomile flowers (available in health-food stores) to the water before boiling. European cosmeticians believe that camomile has a curative, soothing effect on the skin and helps to clean it. If your skin reacts negatively to this treatment by becoming dry and sensitive, forget it, or steam your face gently by applying a compress made by dipping a washcloth in hot water and then wringing it out. Some women with oily or acned skins can steam their faces every day with good effects. Rinse with cool water after steaming.

COMPLEXION BRUSH. I have always used a complexion brush, or a small, natural-bristle brush sold under that name, once every two weeks. This was a practice taught me by my German mother, who uses different brushes on various parts of her body and has fabulous skin. I lather the brush with a mild soap and gently brush my skin with it, starting with the forehead and moving it around my entire face. I work with a circular motion, cleansing small areas at a time. Afterward, my face feels totally clean, firm-skinned and fresh. I only brush my face once every two weeks; if I use the brush more often, it either irritates my skin or seems to have no effect. After I use the brush I rinse it thoroughly, oil it with Nivea oil to keep it soft, and store it in an airtight plastic container to protect it from bacteria. A more modern version of the complexion brush is a polyester fiber sponge called a Buf-Puf. This sponge has a rough surface which virtually seems to sandpaper the skin smooth. It sounds unpleasant, but when used regularly it keeps both oily and dry skin exceptionally smooth and clear. The Buf-Puf can be used every day, once your skin becomes accustomed to it. Both the Buf-Puf and the complexion brush should be used gently.

Skin Care
157

ASTRINGENTS, FRESHENERS, AND CLARIFYING LO-
TIONS. These are alcohol-based lotions which help the
skin shed excess cells, temporarily close pores, and bring
color to the complexion. If your skin is dry, a freshener,
which has less alcohol, is the best toner; pat it on with a
cotton pad. Oily or blemished skins benefit more from astringents and clarifying lotions, which should be wiped
on with a cotton pad. Alcohol-based lotions should be
shaken before use to distribute their ingredients evenly.

MOISTURIZING THE FACE

The face's moisturizing fountains are the blood vessels, which bring a supply of water to the cells. Creams
and moisturizers applied to the skin do not add moisture
per se but merely prevent the water our bodies provide
from escaping. Although this sealing function is the main
role of a cream, cosmetic companies are constantly trying
to convince us with elaborate advertising campaigns that
creams remove wrinkles and make us look younger.

There is no cream on earth, alas, that can actually
remove a wrinkle once it has formed. Creams do soften
the appearance of wrinkles and tend to fill out fine lines,
which look more pronounced minus a moisturizer.
Creams also lubricate the skin, making it softer to the
touch, and protect it from harsh environmental factors.
Therefore, all cosmetologists recommend that if we have
dry or fragile skin, we keep some form of cream on it at
all times—a light, moisturizing lotion for the day and a
heavier, oilier cream at night. In my opinion, some moisturizing agent should always be used around the eyes,
whatever your age or skin type, because the eye area has

no oil glands of its own. This eye cream should be light-textured. Don't forget to cream your neck.

What cream to choose

Dermatologists say that all moisturizing agents are basically the same and serve the same purpose—to lubricate the skin and prevent its natural water from evaporating into the air. The cosmetics industry, on the other hand, fervently tries to sell us elaborate and expensive creams containing exotic ingredients guaranteed to rejuvenate the skin—organic substances such as strawberries and cucumbers, hormones, precious turtle and mink oils, and so on. All these ingredients, dermatologists argue, are useless additives which the skin cannot absorb, and which wouldn't do any good if it could; they say that Crisco is as effective a lubricant and moisturizer as any expensive cream. Do you believe it? More important, do you want to?

Those of us who are penny-wise and practical will instantly resort to Crisco, while those with higher hopes and greater imaginations will stick to their search for the century's wrinkle-removing wonder. Consider that, whatever the hard facts, there is a positive psychological lift to smoothing on a beautifully packaged, divinely scented and textured cream which you firmly believe may make you young again. Fooling yourself is not all bad. Some fine creams, I think, seem to blend well with the skin, giving it a delightfully smooth touch to the fingertips. If you believe in buying expensive creams, do stop yourself long enough to ask the cosmetician behind the counter exactly what ingredient in the pricey concoction is supposed to remove wrinkles, and how. If she has no answer at all, don't waste your money on the cream. Try a sample if you can.

Personally, I believe my skin becomes immune to the same cream and I like to surprise it with different moisturizers. I am always experimenting. I vacillate between the most expensive cream on the market and good old Crisco, which I have mixed in my blender with sweeter-smelling products with great success. I also find after-sun lotions make excellent, light moisturizing creams.

Moisturizing with water

Many famous beauties spray their faces with mineral water, which they believe moisturizes the skin. I advise buying a humidifier for your home, particularly if you live in an arid climate or if your house has central heating. The fine spray of moisture emitted by the humidifier will do much to combat the drying effects of your radiator. A pan of water, on or near the heating duct, will serve as an inexpensive substitute.

MOISTURIZING BODY SKIN

I believe that the best moisturizing agent for body skin is Nivea oil. I use a larger version of the complexion brush (natural bristles, like a back brush) to brush the oil into the skin of my arms, legs, and torso. My skin looks pink and tender afterward, but I have found this method excellent for smoothing away rough skin. A Buf-Puf is also a good smoothing device for feet, elbows, and knees.

Before a party or important occasion most of us have the desire to perform some special psychic or physical ritual that will prepare our faces for the event. A facial treatment leaves the skin with a shinier gloss than ordinary cleansing does. Though this "new" skin is admittedly temporary, it establishes a good base for makeup and gives an important psychic lift when we face our mirrors before going out. The better we believe we look, the more open and confident an image we present to others. The following Ruth Jody Facial is one I developed myself. It will provide you with a relaxed body and mind, as well as with a radiant skin.

1. Do the Body Exercises for Your Face at the end of chapter 4, or at least two or three of them.

2. Deep-clean the skin with a complexion brush. If you have the time and inclination, you may want to steam your face with a camomile sauna afterward.

3. Apply a masque. These paste or gel-like substances tighten the pores and take excess debris with them when they are removed. By not allowing the face to breathe, they prevent the evaporation of the skin's moisture while they are on, plumping it up and giving it a refreshed appearance.

Many people like to make their own masques. You can use the white of an egg—a thin, drying masque—or the yolk, which supposedly imparts proteins, or even some cooked, cooled oatmeal, which firms and softens the skin. I personally prefer to buy a masque. When I am trying to make myself beautiful and relax, I hardly want to put on an apron and start slopping around in the kitchen with my egg

Skin Care
161

beater. I enjoy opening an elegant jar and applying a nicely homogenized, fine-scented product, already made, to my skin. Choose a masque which relates to your skin type—gel or cream based for dry skins, clay based for oily skins.

4. Lie down and put your feet up. Apply cotton pads soaked with witch hazel to your eyelids; this will relax your eyes and cool them. Breathe deeply from your inner being. Visualize a lovely natural scene and concentrate on it—green meadows, a white beach. Don't think about the party, how you're going to look, or last-minute chores you should be doing. Remain in this position for ten or fifteen minutes.

5. Clean off the masque thoroughly with luke-warm water or peel it off, depending on the instructions. Apply a freshener or witch hazel to tone, then moisturizer and makeup.

This ritual should take approximately half an hour. If you have less time, eliminate steps 1 and 2.

MAKEUP FOR THE MATURE FACE

I have never worn much makeup. I don't feel like myself in lipstick and eyeshadow, but like a mask of myself. Recently, however, I engaged a makeup artist to design my face for a party—just as an experiment. I was astounded at how different, how elegant and lovely I looked. Even my elevator man was beside himself with compliments.

I think there is a lesson for everyone to learn from my experience. Too often we have preconceptions about makeup which determine the way our eyes see our faces in the mirror. Many women at forty or fifty use the same color and style of makeup they used at twenty. This dates them as accurately as an outfit from another decade. Some women may also apply makeup clumsily, with too heavy or too light a hand. Others buy whatever shade of makeup fashion magazines tell them is in for the season, without considering how it actually looks on their face. I had obviously been wearing makeup that did not blend with the colors of my skin and hair and applying it badly, which is why I disliked it.

I believe that as we get older we should take advantage of the color and refinement makeup can add to our faces and employ a variety of products with skill and care, but the total effect should be of less rather than more makeup. Nothing to my mind makes a wrinkle look more like a wrinkle than piling layers of heavy pancake and powder over it. Pasty lipstick or lipstick that does not conform to the contours of the lips should be out for every face, but especially for the older one. I also think false eyelashes, vivid green and blue eyeshadows, and rouge which makes the cheeks glow with an iridescent shimmer are unattractive on mature faces.

Try applying a thin, liquid foundation with a moist sponge. Experts tell us that sponging on foundation gives it a clear, translucent look and blends it with the skin. Darker blemishes can then be covered with a thicker concealing cream. In Europe, chic middle-aged women tend to wear eyeshadows in smoky shades of gray, mauve, and brown instead of vivid colors that seem to emphasize the effects of aging on the eyes. Cream rouges in earthy tones are subtle and flattering to the older face.

Take an objective look in the mirror or ask the advice of close friends. If you conclude that your makeup is not flattering and feel incapable of designing a new cosmetic look for yourself, put your face in the hands of an expert. Most major cosmetic companies employ makeup artists who are available where the cosmetics are sold. Ask one to explain what products are used and why and how to apply them. Remember, when in doubt use less. Heavy makeup may look fine when you leave your home, but after several hours outdoors or at a crowded party, it tends to droop, become slick and heavy, and reveal rather than conceal your age.

A WORD ABOUT COSMETICS AND PERFUMES

It is true that the extravagant prices of many cosmetics are all in the packaging and advertising and that the ingredients themselves are worth only pennies. Many experts advise us to buy dime-store cosmetics, because they are basically the same as their well-advertised, costly counterparts. I feel that the more expensive brands of lipstick, eyeshadow, and makeup base are often the sheerest and most subtly colored. If you can afford them, try them. Be sure to test colors on your face and not on the back of your hand, which is totally different in skin tone. I think it's helpful to develop a working vocabulary of cosmetic ingredients (all books on cosmetics supply you with one) and to find out what your cosmetics and skin-care products contain. The FDA now requires cosmetic companies to list ingredients on the package. Know what you are buying.

Many brands of cosmetics cost more because they contain expensive perfumes. Nothing enhances bodily allure more than a marvelous scent. Unfortunately, all of us use innumerable cosmetic products with varying scents that war with one another. Hair rinse, shampoo, makeup base, skin cream, moisturizer, nail polish, and deodorant all smell like something and together or separately may turn noses away. A smell you may find innocuous may revolt someone close to you. I advise friends to buy their basic cosmetic products unscented, if possible. Hypoallergenic cosmetics have little or no perfume, and some shampoos, hair rinses, and creams have lighter scents than others. Allow an expensive and carefully selected perfume to provide your body's dominant aroma. You may want to skip perfume altogether and derive your cologne from an exquisitely scented soap.

Afterword

You have now read my complete program for maintaining a youthful face and body. I hope this book has encouraged you to realize that aging beautifully is by no means impossible. All of us, I believe, can have attractive faces and bodies for the better part of our lives.

Few people are in really terrible condition. If you were I doubt you would be reading *Facelift Without Surgery* because you wouldn't care how you looked. Like most of us, you are probably a touch overweight and inclined to be lazy when it comes to exercise. The chances are that not all the advice in my book pertains to you. If your chin needs my facial exercises, your waistline may be in perfect shape. If your waistline is larger than you would like, your skin may be taut and clear. Take what you need from my book, and tailor it to your individual personality and life-style. If you want to change your appearance, give your present habits a creative and well-considered analysis. Design a program for yourself which guarantees the changes you need to feel better about the way you look. Remember, although any self-improvement program will require some hard work and sacrifice, you should not devote your entire life to a dreary regimen that you do not enjoy.

At first, all changes are difficult, even when they promise desirable results and personal growth. As we get older, changes become harder to make. I believe that the only way to institute vital changes in your life is to be absolutely compulsive and fanatic when you first start to make them. Design a diet, an exercise program, or both, and persevere, come hell or high water. Don't allow yourself to cop out for any reason. If you rapidly relapse, forget to exercise, or substitute spaghetti for fish in your evening meal, you will find yourself back where you started—physically and psychologically—in no time at all. Changing a diet involves personal discipline which may at first seem akin to torture. Face it!

On the other hand, an exercise program—for body or face—involves changing your use of time. You must substitute your new activities for something you did before. Analyze your day carefully. What are you doing that is neither enjoyable nor necessary? Are you having long, dull, repetitive telephone conversations with friends? Are you spending unnecessary time doing household chores? Are you going to movies you really don't enjoy? There are vacant time slots in everyone's day—find yours and make use of them.

Once you make a diet or exercise program an integral part of your existence, you will cease to contemplate these regimens with loathing. Facial exercises may seem silly and tedious, but if you do them I guarantee your feelings, as well as your face, will change. The same goes for regular physical exercise. There are many personal tasks we perform which we take entirely for granted because we know they make us look and feel better. None of us, for example, resents washing our face, or moans, "My God, I have to brush my teeth." Good diet and proper exercise will eventually take the same matter-of-fact role in your life, if you practice them long enough.

Don't be disappointed if you can't be compulsive forever; you shouldn't even try. After three months of doing facial exercises every day, you can afford to skip a day or two when you must. After six months of a strict diet, an éclair will not devastate your figure. Strange as it may sound to you now, once you've stuck to a successful diet or exercise program and reaped the results, lassitude and éclairs will be less of a temptation. Occasional vacations may make you appreciate your regimen, and vice versa.

When you are invited to an important dinner party and simply cannot make your exercise class, you will not secretly rejoice, "Oh, goodie, I won't have to exercise tonight"; instead, you will feel that you're missing something. When you eat an éclair instead of strawberries for dessert, it will taste both marvelous and less marvelous than you imagined. You will enjoy it, eat it with an ecstasy heightened by guilt, and feel glad to return to strawberries the following evening. This will happen because you have learned that your diet and your exercise program make you feel and look good. You will appreciate the results and want to keep them. You will have faith in your program and in your changes. When it comes right down to it, most of us would rather look better than lounge in an armchair and munch éclairs.

Beauty, at any age, is more than skin deep. Accepting yourself and your life will help you to age beautifully.

Not surprisingly, self-acceptance and self-improvement go hand in hand. Once you do something definite and positive to improve the way you look and watch it work, you will feel better about yourself. It is easier to accept your wrinkles if you have just made your facial skin taut and reduced your waistline. The changes may be small— but you accomplished them. You will feel in control of your body and your life. Provided your expectations are realistic, you cannot disappoint yourself. You may never see the world's greatest face or figure in the mirror, but as long as what you see is the best possible version of yourself, you will be satisfied.

Satisfaction, in my opinion, is the best cosmetic for anyone. Look forward to the way things are and will be, instead of backward to the way they were. If you enjoy life and accept yourself, your eyes will sparkle, the corners of your lips will turn up instead of down, and the space between your eyebrows will be smooth, not creased with bitter lines. You will look terrific, and as I said before, what does age have to do with it?

Index

Index
173